The OR Management Series

Improving OR Performance

2nd Edition

A compilation of articles from *OR Manager*

Editor
Pat Patterson
Editor, *OR Manager*

Clinical Editor
Judith M. Mathias, MA, RN
Clinical Editor, *OR Manager*

Copyright © 2011, Access Intelligence, LLC

All rights reserved. No part of this book may be reproduced in any form or by any means, electronic or mechanical, including photocopying or by an information storage and retrieval system, without permission from the publisher.

Publisher

Access Intelligence, LLC
4 Choke Cherry Rd, 2nd Floor
Rockville, MD 20850

Library of Congress Catalog Card Number: 2011937404

ISBN: 978-1-885461-49-0

Printed in the USA

Foreword

OR directors and others concerned with the management of the surgical suite are facing major changes in health care. The Affordable Care Act, better know as health care reform, will increase the pressure to manage the OR more efficiently at less cost and at the same time increase patient safety.

OR Manager has interviewed perioperative leaders and other experts to find out how successful surgical services leadership teams have improved their department's performance. Related articles from the past three years are included in this OR Management Series module.

Some of the productivity challenges in the surgical suite have been around a long time—late starts, inaccurate case times, out-of-date preference cards, and long turnover times. Today, OR managers have data and tools to measure performance and to take action—dashboards, benchmarking, and Lean management.

As in an automobile, dashboards give you data you need to track your progress. Benchmarking can be used to measure your department's performance and compare it with other like facilities. Lean management, based on the principle that small incremental changes routinely applied and sustained over a period of time can result in significant improvement, is helping many ORs achieve their improvement goals. A new approach, Positive Deviance, involves clinicians and staff in solving tough problems that have not responded to traditional approaches.

The good news is that entire team of leaders—nurses, surgeons, anesthesia providers, and staff—are realizing that they have a role in improving OR performance and are joining in collaborative efforts. Team efforts are more likely to succeed.

Performance improvement is an ongoing part of managing the OR. Articles in this module address efficiencies, dashboards, governance, Lean, preference cards, the preoperative process, scheduling, and turnover time.

In this module, you will find ideas and information on improving OR performance that you can use in your surgical suite to keep ahead of changes in health care.

Table of Contents

I. OR Efficiencies 7
   For ORs, More Pressure to Perform 8
   Way to Break Loose From OR Holds 12
   Why are Case-Time Estimates so Often Off? 15
   Is Time on First–Case Starts Well Spent? 17
   What Makes an OR 'Highly Reliable'? 20
   Team Agreement, Competition Boost Record for On-Time Starts 23
   Data Sparks On-Time Improvements 26
   Benchmarking the OR's Key Indicators 28
   Handoffs: What ORs Can Learn From Formula One Race Crews 30
   Looking to Front-Line Clinicians, Staff for Lasting Improvements 33

II. Dashboard and More 39
   OR Dashboards: A Useful Tool for Telling a Story Through Data 40
   Tracking Data, Changing Behavior 43

III. Governance 47
   Is Your OR Leadership Team Up to Health Care Reform Challenges? 48
   OR Governance Builds a Strong Foundation 51

IV. Lean in the OR 55
   Lean Project Helps to Revitalize an SPD 56
   A Lean Process for OR Technology 59

V. Physician Preference Items 61
   Top Strategies for Juggling Quantity, Cost of Physician Preference Items ...62

VI: Preoperative Process 67
   How Clinics Help the Preop Process 68
   Automation Ends Preop Paper Chase 72

VII. Scheduling 77
   Fine-Tuning the Block Schedule? Now Could Be the Right Time 78
   A Toolkit for Managing Block Scheduling 80
   The Research on OR Time Allocation 82
   Effective Block Scheduling Rests on Fair Policies, Active Management 84
   For Urgent and Emergency Cases, Which One Goes to the OR First? 88
   Managing Urgent Cases with Accountability 91
   Surgical Scheduling: Taking an Important Role to the Next Level 93

VIII. Turnover Time 97
   An Engineer's Eye on Turnover Time 98
   Turnover? Focus on Everything Else 101

I. OR Efficiencies

For ORs, More Pressure to Perform

How health care reform will affect hospitals and other facilities will be unfolding for years. There will be some time to prepare. Under the sweeping reform law passed in March 2010, the major expansion in insurance coverage won't take effect until 2014.

The Congressional Budget Office estimates the reform legislation will reduce the number of uninsured by 32 million in 2019. Many of the newly covered will enroll under Medicaid, while others will be able to purchase coverage through new health insurance exchanges.

For hospitals, the prospects are decidedly mixed. Some say hospitals will be winners, but others think that's too optimistic. Though hospitals agreed to give up $155 billion in Medicare funding over the next decade as part of the negotiations to pass the legislation, they expect to make up at least $170 billion by treating fewer uninsured patients, according to Kaiser Health News. But many of the newly insured will be in government programs that don't pay well.

A few realities

Reform is likely to be an extension of what has been happening for years, at least on the payment side, says Nathan Kaufman of Kaufman Strategic Advisors LLC, San Diego. The government has squeezed Medicare payments for nearly a decade and will continue to do so. Medicaid enrollment has grown during the recession as unemployment has risen, yet 39 states are freezing or cutting Medicaid payments to providers.

A few realities he cites:
- More than half of community hospitals' revenue is from public programs, including Medicare and Medicaid.
- Community hospitals lose 15 cents of every dollar they spend caring for Medicare patients.
- 300 to 500 more baby boomers reach Medicare age every hour.

There are also new realities. Hospitals will see some of their payments put at risk in the coming years through a new value-based purchasing plan and penalties for hospital-acquired conditions and readmissions.

Pressure for performance

The economic picture will create more pressure than ever for OR performance.

"The pressure exists to improve perioperative performance because that is 65% of a hospital's bottom line," says Jeff Peters, president of Surgical Directions, LLC, a Chicago-based consulting firm. "There is tremendous pressure on hospitals to improve the bottom-line, and they look to the OR to be a major contributor to that."

Also in the forefront—quality and accountabil-

Hospital payment-to-cost ratios, 1988-2008

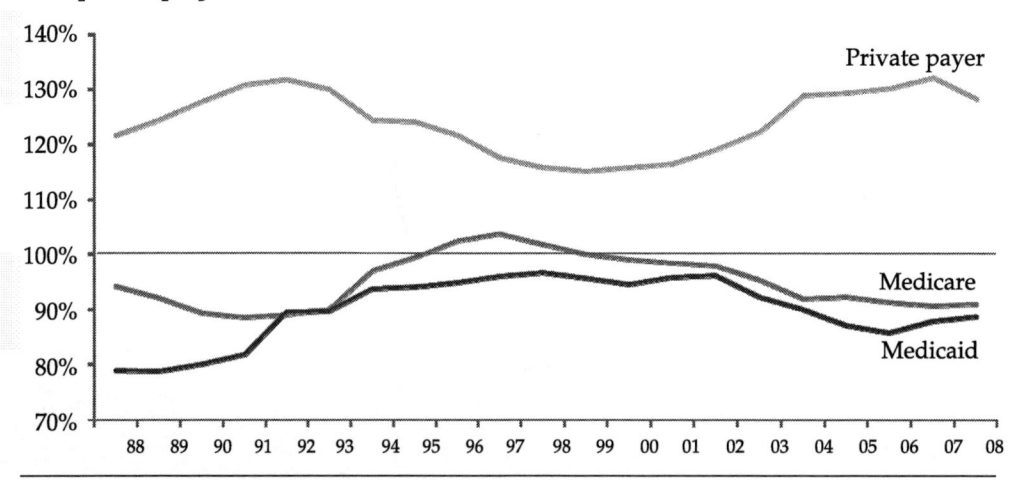

Source: American Hospital Association Annual Survey data, 2008, for community hospitals.
Medicaid includes Medicaid Disproportionate Share payments.

Hospital physician-generated revenue

Net annual revenue per hospital per physician from referrals, tests, and procedures performed at the hospital.

Neurosurgery	$2.8 million
General surgey	$2.1 million
Orthopedic surgery	$2.1 million
Gastroenterology	$1.5 million
Urology	$1.4 million

Source: Merritt Hawkins, 2010. www.merritthawkins.com

---

ity. The reform legislation has initiatives aimed at improving quality while lowering costs.

"OR throughput will be important," adds Kaufman, "but so will the total cost of the patient episode and patient satisfaction—we may eventually be rewarded or punished based on patient satisfaction scores from Medicare."

Though the prospects seem daunting, Kaufman says it's no different from the challenges any industry faces. "You are expected to produce better products at a lower cost at a certain price point—that eventually is what ORs are going to be expected to do.

"The way you do that," he continues, "is to identify best practice protocols; eliminate variability and waste; use data for developing and monitoring your protocols; and look at your processes to see if there are opportunities to eliminate steps, duplication, and unnecessary use of expensive supplies."

A focus on the fundamentals

Where should perioperative leaders place their efforts? The response from consultants OR Manager interviewed was unanimous—focus on the fundamentals. Peters emphasizes these priorities:

1. Reinforce good OR governance.
2. Find ways to grow surgical volume.
3. Increase OR performance so you can expand services with the same resources.
4. Lower costs, particularly for supplies.

(Suggested strategies are in the sidebar, p 10.)

Reinforce good OR governance

Better performance starts with a strong governance structure. Three criteria for good governance were outlined by Randy Heiser, president and CEO of Sullivan Healthcare Consulting, Ann Arbor, Michigan:

- physician leadership
- constant communication with the medical staff
- support for the leadership team that goes all the way to the CEO.

Physician leadership is an essential element. "I have yet to find an effective governance structure that didn't have physician leaders," he says.

Physician leadership is not the same as physician control, Heiser cautions. Physician leadership is being willing to tell a surgeon that doing a particular case at 2 am is not appropriate. In contrast, "being afraid to do the right thing because a physician might react badly is physician control."

A strong multidisciplinary leadership group can develop surgical scheduling policies that can be reinforced for all members of the surgical team. Regular, consistent communication is needed to convey, explain, and reinforce the scheduling policies and other rules, Heiser adds. And those policies will hold up only if the organization's senior leadership is willing to stand behind the OR leadership team.

Beef up the business side

The principles of good supply and inventory management are well known—keep preference cards updated, strive for standardization, manage custom packs, put every possible product on consignment, capture charges, and so on.

One of the best investments an OR can make is to hire a business manager, a position Heiser calls "a CFO for surgery."

"This is one of the most cost-effective positions you can create. I would say that in 9 out of 10 clients where we have recommended that position, it has paid for itself in 3 months."

He suggests that the position is most successful if the business manager is recruited from a related department, such as finance or materials management, so the person is already familiar with the business side of health care.

Expect to see more employed physicians

Health care economics are causing a shift in the hospital-physician relationship, with implications for the OR. More physicians are seeking to be employed by hospitals and health systems.

Among forces driving physician employment are uncertainty about the economic climate, declining reimbursement, increasing practice overhead, and in some states, the malpractice environment.

Improving OR performance

Strategies offered by Jeff Peters of Surgical Directions, LLC.

Develop a collaborative OR governance structure

Effective management of the OR schedule and scheduling policies requires a multidisciplinary leadership team that involves surgeon, anesthesia, and nurse leadership. Involving the hospital's senior leadership, ideally the CEO, ensures that the team has the authority to set and enforce policy.

Move to 8-hour blocks

Aim to provide surgeons with 8-hour blocks and require 75% utilization.

Eight-hour blocks allow surgeons who work at the facility regularly to start in the morning and operate continuously through the day without gaps, which is efficient both for the surgeon and facility.

A related rule: Leave 20% of rooms open each day so surgeons without an 8-hour block have access to OR time.

Have patients ready for surgery

Having patients ready for surgery minimizes delays and cancellations because of clinical issues or missing paperwork.

Refine the preadmission process so that as much as possible, 90% of patients' charts are complete 3 days before surgery, and 95% are complete the day before.

Consider specialty teams

For high-volume specialties, consider specialty teams of nursing personnel. Some facilities include anesthesiologists and nurse anesthetists on the teams. Specialty teams reduce variability because they know the surgeons' routines and setups. Teams can create a balancing act for staffing, however.

Tighten up on supply management

Reinforce basic concepts:
- Do you capitalize surgical supplies as you buy them (ie, consider them an asset), or do you immediately expense them? Converting supplies into an asset can give you a one-time gain of $50,000 to $100,000 per OR.
- Make sure that implants and any other eligible supplies are placed on consignment.
- Review par levels to make sure the right supply quantities are available but not overstocked.

Review staffing

Some ORs still use traditional 8-hour shifts when staggered and flexible shifts would be more cost-effective.

If, as in many facilities, more cases are being performed between 5 and 7 pm, stagger staffing through the day so those hours can be covered without paying overtime. Make sure staffing doesn't drop off too rapidly after 3 pm.

"We are beginning to see more surgeons think of employment as a means to stabilize their incomes," Kaufman says.

The Medical Group Management Association reports that hospital employment among its physician members rose to 37% in 2009 from 25% in 2003.

Physicians bring hospitals a lot of revenue, with a specialist generating on average $1.8 million in net revenue a year, according to the recruiting firm Merritt Hawkins (chart, p 8).

In another development, many hospitals are looking to buy ambulatory surgery centers (ASCs) from their physician owners and convert them into hospital outpatient departments because hospital-based outpatient surgery provides higher reimbursement than in an ASC, according to Becker's ASC Review published by Scott Becker of McGuireWoods. Medicare pays hospitals substantially more than ASCs for the same procedures, and the gap is often greater with commercial payers, Becker says.

Pressure to perform

What should OR directors know about the shifting economic climate for physicians?

"Physicians are coming to realize they need to be more efficient than ever before," comments Bryan Warren of Accelero, a consulting firm owned by Zimmer that focuses on management of the orthopedic service line. Warren says he recently talked with a surgeon who said that if he doesn't find a way to perform more joint procedures in less time, he doesn't want to do the surgery anymore because it doesn't pay well enough.

Will better alignment ensue?

Don't assume that because surgeons are employed, closer collaboration with OR leaders will automatically follow, Warren cautions.

"Employment is an alignment strategy," he says, "but it does not ensure alignment in and of itself. When surgeons walk into the OR, they don't think of themselves as employees. They still have a certain amount of autonomy in the way they function."

Warren adds: "Strategies that allow the OR to run better to meet the needs of the physicians are probably more important than ever, regardless of whether the physicians are employed or not."

He echoed the advice about good OR governance, saying that the physicians need to be actively engaged in governance, setting goals, and reinforcing policies.

Reaching out

Warren notes that he does see physicians reaching out to hospitals in a more collaborative manner than in the past, and "We are telling hospitals to take advantage of that."

Hospitals that employ surgeons should build in administrative responsibilities, he advised, so they are required to take an active leadership role.

Physicians who are not employed are sometimes offered incentives in the form of medical director positions or comanagement agreements, in which there is a formal arrangement between the hospital and physician to share management of a service line.

Warren says his firm is receiving a lot of inquiries about comanagement.

"In some cases it's a good idea," he says. "In others, you can accomplish the same thing without all the work it takes to put that together. In our mind, it's one of a number of solutions."

A greater urgency

No matter what lies ahead, perioperative leaders will face more urgency in the areas they already focus on: patient safety and quality, throughput, and cost. Take the opportunity to diagnosis your current situation and plan a strategy, suggests Ryan Bengtson of the Huron Consulting Group, Chicago.

Three areas to focus on:
- Actionable data. Can your information system produce the reports you need for making decisions?
- Operational effectiveness. Do a diagnosis: What is your current OR utilization? How well are you using the OR facilities and staff you have?
- Reinforce your governance structure. Strong leadership will be critical.

This is not just an OR committee that meets every month or two, Bengtson advises. He suggests asking: What is your leadership structure for monitoring and measuring systems, providing feedback, and resolving disputes? Do you have the right mix of nurses, surgeons, and anesthesia personnel, and other leaders involved? Are there clear expectations and individual accountability?

OR leaders already know the fundamentals—improving through put allocating and managing OR time efficiently, and relentlessly working to improve performance while conserving resources. Success is in the execution. ❖

—*Pat Patterson*

References

Iglehart J. Historic passage—Reform at last. *N Engl J Med*. Posted March 24, 2010.

Kaiser Family Foundation. White House/Congressional Leadership Reconciliation Bill Health Care and Education Reconciliation Act of 2010 (H.R. 4872): Summary of Coverage Provisions. www.kff.org

This article originally appeared in OR Manager, *May 2010;26:6-9.*

Way to Break Loose From OR Holds

OR holds slow the entire hospital's throughput. "What happens in the OR doesn't stay in the OR—it affects the whole system," says Christy Dempsey, RN, MBA, CNOR, senior vice president of clinical operations for PatientFlow Technology, Inc, Boston.

The emergency department (ED) and ICU are particularly hard hit.

Holds can cause OR cancellations, delayed admissions, and unhappy staff due to overtime. All this adds up to money.

Avoiding bottlenecks in the OR requires dissecting the complexity of holds, working through a team with the power to refine processes, and using technology to help. First, you need to understand what causes OR holds, and then your team can develop strategies to address the issues.

Realities of OR holds

Why do OR holds occur? The answer might surprise you, as it did Tammy Straub, RN, MSN, CNOR, director of perioperative services at Lehigh Valley Hospital.

Straub advises OR managers not to assume causes of holds but to gather data first. She used data analysis to dispel several common theories for OR holds – not enough PACU beds to accommodate postoperative patients; too many OR procedures ending at the same time, leading to surges based on acuity; and lack of PACU staff. Although sometimes too many patients in the PACU were waiting for inpatient beds, this, too, had a weak effect on OR holds. Instead, staffing patterns in the PACU needed to change to meet patients' care needs, and real-time monitoring of bed status was needed.

Dempsey, who has consulted with many ORs, says variability in the elective OR schedule is the number one reason for OR holds: "It has the biggest impact on hospital census." Research by Eugene Litvak, PhD, and his colleagues from Boston University supports this, showing that nearly 70% of diversions from the ICU were associated with variability in scheduled OR time. When elective surgery peaked, so did diversions.

Here are some strategies to help you determine causes of holds and develop solutions that fit your needs.

Form the best team

Taking time to select the right team members will save you time in the long run.

"Get the right people on the bus," says Straub. "Have people who want a positive end result."

In addition to PACU and OR leadership and staff representation, other team members should include the chief of anesthesiology, a surgeon (if you cannot find a surgeon to serve, be sure to keep surgeons informed of your progress), patient logistics (bed management) staff, a representative from the preop area, and a nursing supervisor. Straub says it's also important to support the team with resources, particularly a person who can analyze data.

Define the problem

The team needs to define and track OR holds. After data analysis showed a hold time of 913 hours (equal to about 300 laparoscopic cholecystectomies) in one fiscal year, Straub knew she needed to act. First, nurses simply marked hold times on a calendar; later they developed a form to document reasons for the holds. This information can be retrieved from the hospital's information system.

To ensure consistent data collection, it's important to define hold time. Lehigh Valley defines a short hold as 15 minutes or less, and it's usually not significant; a long hold is anything beyond 15 minutes. Here is where to concentrate your efforts.

As you begin to develop solutions, align yourself with other hospital initiatives rather than reinvent the wheel. For example, Lehigh Valley's team used the model of their ED's paging alert system to create one of their own.

Be proactive

The best strategy, of course, is to resolve situations before an OR hold occurs.

"The key piece is to deal proactively with external and internal barriers to ensure efficient, yet safe flow of patients," says Mary Jane Neri, RN, MSN, administrative manager, Beaumont Hospital, Royal Oak, Michigan. Neri says close collaboration among PACU, OR, and preop area staff is key, along with keeping a close eye on multiple factors such as number of PACU beds and mix of inpatients and outpatients.

A good person to keep a close eye is the PACU charge nurse. At Lehigh Valley, the position is rotated among a cadre of nurses who have been selected and trained for the position to ensure consistency.

PACU nurses interested in being a charge nurse apply and are interviewed by a committee of staff nurses and the patient care coordinator. The nurse receives an educational packet and works with another charge nurse for 1 month.

"Nurses view these as empowering, leadership positions," says Straub, noting there is no associated pay differential.

One duty of the PACU charge nurse is to assess and adjust assignments. PACU patients require differing nurse-patient ratios depending on where they are in the recovery process. According to the American Society of PeriAnesthesia Nurses standards, the nurse-patient ratio should be no higher than 1:2 for Phase I, 1:3 for Phase II, and 1:3 to 1:5 for extended observation.

The higher nurse-patient ratio can be a hard sell to staff. Straub says she and her team focused on the benefits for patients and made reducing OR hold time a goal for everyone on the perioperative team. An added benefit was a lasting partnership between the OR and PACU.

PACU charge nurses also determine readiness for transfer and serve as the hub of communication by keeping the major players for patient flow informed: PACU staff, OR charge nurse, patient logistics staff, lead anesthesia provider, and charge nurses on key inpatient units.

"The charge nurse is the traffic cop and doesn't recover patients," says Pam Cipriano, RN, PhD, FAAN, chief clinical officer and chief nursing officer at the University of Virginia Health System (UVHS) in Charlottesville, Virginia. "This allows decision making on a patient-by-patient basis." Charge nurses may help out at the bedside with procedures such as reintubations or placing patients on an ECG monitor.

An electronic bed status system that gives real-time information will help you to be proactive, as can a bed-planning team, such as the one UVHS uses. The team, which includes the patient logistics area and units that routinely experience capacity issues, meets daily for 15 minutes in mid-afternoon for a planning session.

As Lehigh Valley did, examine your staffing pattern in the PACU. You may find you don't need more staff but rather need to realign staff so they are available at peak times. Consider other staffing resources, too. Neri says at Beaumont Hospital, nurses in the preop area care for patients who have been recovered in PACU and are waiting for beds. If necessary, the orthopedic unit provides additional staff to the preop area. UVHS set a standard requiring environmental services to complete all bed turnovers in 60 minutes or less.

Be creative when it comes to space. Cipriano says part of the PACU serves as a satellite ICU when demand is high; critical care float staff care for these patients.

Cipriano recommends identifying "artificial barriers" slowing the flow of patients. "For example, we've reoriented staff so that if a nurse who will be taking care of a patient can't take report from the PACU, someone else does." The PACU nurse provides a face-to-face update when the patient arrives on the unit.

Use technology

Developing a staged alert system, such as the one at Lehigh Valley, can help avoid holds and promote quick response should one occur. Alerts range from 0 (standard operating procedure) to 4 (OR hold is occurring) and are transmitted by an intranet paging system. The charge nurse pages several people at once, including the nurse supervisor on duty, senior administration, charge nurses on key inpatient units, and a patient flow coordinator, who serves as the liaison between patient logistics and clinical staff.

"The pagers allow us to give specific information like 'I need 5 female beds,'" says Straub. The real-time communication also cuts down delays due to back-and-forth questions between PACU and patient logistics. Lehigh Valley uses a grid listing actions for each resource person at each alert stage so there are no questions as to who does what.

The alert system, added to other strategies, helped the hospital reduce hold minutes by an impressive 75% in 1 year.

UVHS uses another technology option: wireless voice communication.

"It improves the speed and ease of contact between OR and PACU staff," says Cipriano. The system facilitates conferencing between, for example, the central nursing office, patient logistics, and the PACU charge nurse.

Discharge patients on time

Cipriano says an important factor in avoiding OR holds is inpatient discharge by noon.

"If we have 50% of patients out by noon it gives us the flexibility to move patients," she says. "When we have less than that, we have patient backups that ultimately affect the OR."

Planning for discharge begins within 24 hours of admission. Physicians are encouraged to write discharge orders the day before or by 9 am the day the patient is to leave the hospital. These steps provide time to coordinate resources and activate specific discharge pathways such as ones for the pharmacy and laboratory. Incentives for early discharge include financial support for resident and nursing education programs.

Cipriano says timely discharge and other strategies have reduced OR holds by one-third from 3 years ago, and the length of holds has decreased significantly.

Smooth your schedule

If your OR schedule has peaks on certain days

of the weeks, smoothing the OR schedule may be for you. Dempsey of PatientFlow Technology explains that if, for example, total joint replacements are performed only on Tuesday and Wednesday, inpatient beds on the units receiving these postoperative patients are then full for that length of stay. Patients who arrive in the ED don't have access to beds on the appropriate units, so they are sent to other units or are kept in the ED or PACU until a bed is ready.

"You need to reduce artificial variability," she says. To do that, separate scheduled and unscheduled cases and analyze elective block utilization, defined as the case time within the blocks (patient in to patient out of the OR room plus turnover time) divided by the available block time. This will show you how usage needs to be adjusted.

Dempsey says changing a surgeon's schedule may not be as difficult as you think. "A relatively small group of surgeons working with the manager can make things happen. Surgeons need to be at the table and make decisions, not just give input."

Having the surgeons set and enforce the rules keeps OR managers out of the middle. You don't necessarily need the "titled" surgeons, such as the chief of surgery, on the committee.

"The best way is to have high-volume, relatively vocal surgeons who want to make a difference and are credible with their peers," says Dempsey.

Hospitals need to have services such as physical therapy available on the weekends and to adjust staffing in the PACU to match staff to demand.

Celebrate successes

OR holds should be discussed in every team meeting in all perioperative areas. As you see OR hold time fall and throughput improve, Straub and Leader suggest sharing success stories with staff and letting them know how much you appreciate their efforts as a team. ❖

—*Cynthia Saver, RN, MS*

References

Dempsey C. Smooth the elective OR schedule? A large hospital makes it happen. *OR Manager*. 2006;22(4):1-6.

McManus M L, Long M C, Cooper A, et al. Variability in surgical caseload and access to intensive care services. *Anesthesiology*. 2003;98(6):1491-1496.

McGowan, J E, Truwit, J D, Cipriano P, et al. Operating room efficiency and hospital capacity: factors affecting operating room use during maximum hospital census. *J Am Coll Surg*. 2007;204:865-872.

This article originally appeared in OR Manager, *March 2008;24:14-15.*

Why are Case-Time Estimates so Often Off?

You've no doubt worked hard on turnover time and on-time starts to improve your OR's performance. But there's a factor you may be overlooking—the accuracy of your case-duration estimates.

These estimates have a big impact. Underestimate case times, and cases run over. Then subsequent cases either start late, or you have to scramble to find another room. But if you overestimate times, cases end early, leaving awkward gaps in the middle of the day. Surgeons and patients have to be asked to move up to fill the gaps. It can feel like crisis management, and it drives down patient, physician, and staff satisfaction.

The OR Benchmarks Collaborative (ORBC), analyzing 12 months of data for a sample of 72 subscribers with 1.3 million cases submitted, found that with targeted efforts, subscribers were able to improve case-duration accuracy by an average of 3%. They were also able to make improvements of 3.2% in subsequent-case start-time accuracy, 5.1% in prime-time utilization, and 8% in both surgical case volume and case minutes.

Over the first 20 months of the collaborative, subscribers in general have improved case-time accuracy by 29% using the collaborative's tools. Overestimated time fell by 12%, and underestimates decreased by 33%. The ORBC tools enable managers to analyze a great deal of data quickly and easily. ORBC is a partnership between OR Manager, Inc, and McKesson that provides a web-based dashboard on key performance indicators and analytical tools (www. orbenchmarking.com).

Why are estimates inaccurate?

OR directors often scratch their heads about why case-duration estimates are off, says Tina Foster, RN, MBA, CNOR, of McKesson Business Performance Solutions. Automated OR scheduling systems typically compute average case durations for each type of procedure each surgeon performs. In general, the system considers the surgeon's past 10 to 15 cases for each procedure, discards the longest and shortest times, and averages the times in between.

Foster says there are 4 major reasons why estimates are inaccurate:
• Procedure files have multiple names for the same procedure.
• Cases involving multiple procedures, which take more time, are counted in with times for a single procedure.
• Default cleanup and setup times are used in scheduling, regardless of the complexity of the procedures.
• Surgeons are allowed to override system-generated times for case duration.

Here's how each factor affects OR operations and suggestions for some solutions.

Keeping procedure files clean

An eroded procedure file is the most common reason for inaccurate case-time estimates.

"Looking into the procedure file, you might find, for example, that laparoscopic cholecystectomy has been posted under a number of different names in the past 6 months, such as lap chole, laparoscopic chole, or lap cholecystectomy," Foster says. When the system figures an average for lap chole, it doesn't know to look under all of those different names. Thus, it doesn't include data for all lap choles performed during the time period in question.

Another problem is uncommon procedures that aren't performed often enough for the data to be representative. When most organizations build their systems, Foster notes, they include a rough estimate for these uncommon procedures and expect enough data to accumulate. But if there aren't enough of those cases, the case duration estimate will be inaccurate.

Procedure files tend to be unruly. For the average community hospital, the best practice for a procedure file is about 2,500 different procedures, she says. But it's not unusual to have 10,000 or 12,000.

Ideally, facilities would use a standardized procedure dictionary for naming and scheduling cases. Most surgical services information systems provide such a dictionary. But many ORs elect to customize the dictionaries, which eventually leads to inconsistent naming.

ORBC, with its data-mining tools, gives subscribers the ability to drill into their case scheduling statistics to identify which procedures or physicians are outliers.

One facility found only about 39% of its case-duration estimates were accurate. Analyzing the data, the facility learned orthopedics was a lower performer than the other service lines, and one high-volume surgeon was a statistical outlier. Examining the data in more detail, they discovered that only his total hip cases, specifically his right total hip cases, were underestimated by about one-half hour. After further investigation, they found his office routinely scheduled all of his total hip procedures as left hip cases. As a result, when a right hip procedure was performed, the staff had to change the room setup, which took about 30 minutes.

"This was driving the performance of the whole OR, not to mention raising quality and safety issues," Foster says.

Accommodating multiple procedures

Multiple procedures are a second factor leading to inaccurate case-duration estimates. For instance, a lap chole is performed with an appendectomy and an oophorectomy. If the case is posted as a lap chole, the case-duration data will go into the lap chole file. It will skew the case-duration statistics because the combined case takes longer than a lap chole alone.

A solution is to provide a method for the scheduler to accommodate cases routinely performed together so the data will be kept separately from the standard procedure file, Foster suggests. There should also be an override process that allows the scheduler to post multiple procedures not often done together so these statistics will also be kept separately.

Accounting for setup and cleanup times

A third factor that throws off case-duration estimates is the way the scheduling system adds time for between-case activities like setup and cleanup. There are a number of ways to handle this, and they can affect the accuracy of estimates, Foster notes.

A common approach is to set up standard "time buckets" to add to the end of each procedure for setup and cleanup. That's the easiest approach, she says, particularly if clerical staff will be doing the scheduling. But it can lead to inaccurate case-duration estimates because actual setup and cleanup times vary considerably by type of procedure. For example, the setup for an appendectomy might take 10 minutes, while a total hip setup might take 45 minutes.

Another common approach is to provide standard setup and cleanup time buckets by 3 levels of case complexity, such as simple, minor, and major. For example, for a simple case, you might add 15 minutes for setup and cleanup; for a minor case, 30 minutes; and for a major case, 45 minutes.

But this approach doesn't take into account situations where cases of different complexity follow one another. For example, an appendectomy is followed by a total hip replacement. If the appendectomy has 15 minutes added at the end, the total hip case will be delayed because there is not enough time for the setup. In the reverse situation, where a total hip case is followed by an appendectomy, there would be 45 minutes before the appendectomy, which would mean downtime.

Although these buckets may seem like the easiest way to allow for between-case activities, "they often don't work well," Foster says. "You can see how stringing 20 to 40 cases together in a day with these mismatched turnover times would lead to an inaccurate schedule and a high degree of dissatisfaction."

A better approach is to add separate setup and cleanup buckets on the front end and back end of the case times. For example, for an appendectomy, you might add 10 minutes on the front end for setup and 5 minutes at the back end for cleanup; with total hip, you might add 30 minutes on the front end, and 15 minutes at the end of the case. Though this system is more accurate, it's more complicated to implement and manage.

"Organizations are starting to use more complex methods because they realize the importance of scheduling accuracy, but it's a hard process—there is no silver bullet," Foster notes.

Surgeons overriding the system

There are 2 variations on system overrides, Foster notes. In private practice settings, a surgeon might say he or she can perform the case in less time than the system reports to fit the case into the time available or to fit more cases into the surgeon's block. When physicians are salaried, they may have an incentive to overbook case times so their schedule looks full, providing them with more free time during the day.

"There should be a process in place that requires scheduled case times to be driven by system estimates. There should also be a clear policy for exceptions that requires approval or documentation," Foster advises. For example, the policy would give recourse to a surgeon who knows a patient has adhesions or another condition that will require additional time. Otherwise, the system-generated time should prevail.

Organizations that invest time and effort to improve their case-time accuracy can make big gains in performance, she says. Being accurate in estimating case times is as important in effective utilization of OR time and customer satisfaction as efforts to improve on-time first-case starts and reduce turnover time. ❖

This article originally appeared in OR Manager, *April 2008;24:21-22.*

Is Time on First-Case Starts Well Spent?

OR leaders spend a great deal of time and effort on improving on-time starts for first cases of the day. Is that time well spent? How can you determine whether reducing late starts would help save substantive costs before you embark on the effort?

Two articles in *Anesthesia & Analgesia* evaluated the psychology and economics of first-case-of-the-day starts. The second article includes a table for doing a quick calculation of potential cost savings (chart below).

Psychology of first-case starts

The psychological study was motivated by an observation that we made at a hospital that had a committee that met for months to improve on-time starts. Many of the physicians and nurse leaders seemed to assume that starting the first case late "cascaded," causing all subsequent cases to be late. When interviewed, however, none knew correctly how the start times of cases that appeared on the schedule were calculated. This observation suggested a psychological bias.

We had an opportunity to explore the psychology of first-case starts when the same hospital used an anonymous electronic survey about preference cards before implementation of a new OR information system. We added some scientific questions to the survey.

For example, we asked the participants to respond to the following statement: "Starting the first case in a room 10 minutes late because of missing supplies likely causes each following case to start at least 10 minutes late." They could respond on a 5-point scale from "strongly disagree" to "strongly agree."

The statement is not true because if cases are scheduled based on the mean of historical data, then slightly more than half of cases take less time than scheduled. At the studied hospital, the cases that followed a first case of the day that started 5 minutes to 15 minutes late did, of course, start on average later than if the first case started on time. But the average increase in tardiness was only 1.1 minutes, not 10 minutes.

Results reveal bias

Respondents had a 1 in 5 (20%) chance to guess the correct answer of "strongly disagree," but only 1 in 57 (2%) did so. When the results for those who answered "disagree" were added, 12% gave the correct answer when there was a 40% chance of guessing right. The results, which were worse than random chance, are precisely what would be expected if staff have a psychological bias that cases either start on time or late (ie, do not start early).

We also evaluated to what extent the respondents knew that fewer than half of cases last longer than scheduled. The knowledge was low, with only 32% answering correctly, which was less than the random rate of 50%. More impor-

Daily reduction in labor cost from reducing first-case-of-the-day tardiness
(normalized to labor cost of $1 per regularly scheduled minute)

	Reduction in tardiness (min)							
	1	2	3	4	5	6	7	8
1	1.1	2.2	3.3	4.4	5.5	6.6	7.7	8.8
2	2.2	4.4	6.6	8.8	11.0	13.2	15.4	17.6
3	3.3	6.6	9.9	13.2	16.5	19.8	23.1	26.4
4	4.4	8.8	13.2	17.6	22.0	26.4	30.8	35.2
5	5.5	11.0	16.5	22.0	27.5	33.0	38.5	44.0
6	6.6	13.2	19.8	26.4	33.0	39.6	46.2	52.8
7	7.7	15.4	23.1	30.8	38.5	46.2	53.9	61.6
8	8.8	17.6	26.4	35.2	44.0	52.8	61.6	70.4
9	9.9	19.8	29.7	39.6	49.5	59.4	69.3	79.2
10	11.0	22.0	33.0	44.0	55.0	66.0	77.0	88.0

Source: Dexter F, Epstein R H. *Anesth Analg.* 2009;108:1282-1287. Reprinted with permission.

tantly, none of the respondents with this knowledge applied it to answering the question about first-case starts correctly. This finding, once again, is consistent with staff having a bias that cases do not start early, even though cases do start early more than half the time when scheduled appropriately.

Results seen in earlier study

We have seen such results before. Previously, we performed an experimental study of case scheduling with nursing students at a different university (Dexter et al, 2007). In that study, everyone had to learn and be tested on their knowledge that around half the cases start early in order to proceed with case scheduling. Just as for the new first-case-start study, that knowledge was ignored.

These results show that education on principles of first-case starts and waiting is likely of no benefit. If we want to reduce waiting times of patients and surgeons, committees will not succeed—and incidentally, neither will improving first-case starts.

Instead, the average lateness of starts is built into the scheduled start-time estimates and patient arrival times (Wachtel and Dexter, 2007 and 2009). Will changing the start-time calculations result in counterproductive changes in behavior? Ironically no; because of the bias, people have essentially no idea how the scheduled start times are chosen.

Minimal economic savings

The advantage of focusing on first-case starts is principally an economic one, but rarely is the focus important economically. Why is this not obvious? In our 2006 systematic review of service-specific staffing calculations (McIntosh, et al), we included the validated methodology for using each hospital's OR information system data or anesthesia group data to calculate the savings from improving first-case starts. The example in that paper showed minimal economic savings from improving on-time starts.

Likely, we know why the results do not seem to apply. In the psychology study, we asked a third question about basic knowledge of OR efficiency (ie, economics of OR staffing). There was a 40% chance to guess the correct answer, and 37% did so. The good news is that there was not a bias, just lack of knowledge. Nevertheless, the result shows that knowledge of OR efficiency appears not to be learned "on the job" by working in ORs. Consequently, referring members of a committee to the 2006 review article is unlikely to be convincing unless they want to learn the science because it would seem not to apply to your own facility.

Determining potential savings

The second new paper includes a table designed to help in determining how much labor-cost savings you could expect from improving on-time starts for first cases of the day. The table is intuitive and can be used with your own data. Understanding the table does not rely on understanding principles of OR efficiency. Note that the table does not include the value of reducing the intangible cost of delayed surgeons and patients. That can be fixed without actually changing the on-time start by planning the average lateness in subsequent scheduled start times (Wachtel and Dexter, 2007 and 2009).

Using the table

To use the table to determine the potential cost savings by reducing tardiness for first cases of the day, select the cell corresponding to the typical number of ORs with more than 8 hours of cases and turnovers and the anticipated reduction in tardiness. Multiply the value in the cell by the actual staffing cost at your facility in dollars per minute.

For example, at the studied 6-OR facility, there were 2 ORs running more than 8 hours of cases each day and a proposed reduction in tardiness of 3 minutes. Therefore, the value in the cell would be 6.6. Based on an OR labor cost of $3.35 per regularly scheduled minute of OR time, a typical value including both nursing and anesthesia costs, the daily savings for the surgical suite would be approximately $22.11, where $22.11 = 6.6 x $3.35.

For a facility that gets a result like $22.11, no more analysis is required because interventions to improve on-time starts will cost more in comparison to changing OR schedules, which usually is a one-time cost of a few hours of programmers' time.

For some facilities with large average lateness of first-case starts and almost all ORs with more than 8 hours of cases, the estimated savings from the table can be far larger. If substantive savings seem possible, then that value should not be considered correct and used to justify an investment. Instead, the next step is to confirm the results by performing the full analysis (McIntosh et al, 2006). ❖

—Franklin Dexter, MD, PhD
University of Iowa
www.FranklinDexter.net

Franklin Dexter, MD, PhD, is a researcher in the science of OR management.

References

Dexter E U, Dexter F, Masursky D, et al. Both bias and lack of knowledge influence organizational focus on first case of the day starts. *Anesth Analg.* 2009;108:1257-1261.

Dexter F, Epstein R H. Typical savings from each minute reduction in tardy first case of the day starts. *Anesth Analg.* 2009;108:1262-1267.

Dexter F, Xiao Y, Dow A J, et al. Coordination of appointments for anesthesia care outside of operating rooms using an enterprise-wide scheduling system. *Anesth Analg.* 2007;105:1701-1710.

McIntosh C, Dexter F, Epstein R H. Impact of service-specific staffing, case scheduling, turnovers, and first-case starts on anesthesia group and operating room productivity: Tutorial using data from an Australian hospital. *Anesth Analg.* 2006;103:1499-1516.

Wachtel R E, Dexter F. Simple method for deciding what time patients should be ready on the day of surgery without procedure-specific data. *Anesth Analg.* 2007;105:127-140.

Wachtel R E, Dexter F. Reducing tardiness from scheduled start times by making adjustments to the operating room schedule. *Anesth Analg.* 2009;108:1902-1909.

This article originally appeared in OR Manager, *January 2010;26:22-24.*

What Makes an OR 'Highly Reliable'?

What makes an organization "highly reliable"—able to avoid the rare but serious breakdowns that can have devastating consequences for patients?

A highly reliable organization is one that is "exceptionally consistent in accomplishing their goals and avoiding potentially catastrophic errors," notes the Agency for Healthcare Research and Quality (AHRQ). Some familiar examples—the airlines, nuclear power, and aircraft carriers.

Becoming "highly reliable" isn't a matter of adopting a new quality improvement method, "roadmap," or checklist, AHRQ cautions. It's a mindset or a culture that is essential for those approaches to work. The goal is to have a "culture and processes that radically reduce system failures" and respond effectively when there is a failure.

The highly reliable OR

What makes a perioperative department highly reliable? Kaiser Permanente's (KP) California regions have introduced Highly Reliable Surgical Teams. Features include a team-based culture and standardized approaches to processes like preoperative verification.

Highly Reliable Surgical Teams have their roots in 2 Kaiser studies. The most recent, published in 2009, found surgical teams with lower scores for team behaviors were linked to worse patient outcomes (sidebar, p 22).

An earlier study, reported in 2003, one of the first to investigate the effect of preoperative briefings, found briefings were associated with better staff morale, reduced nurse turnover, and improved staff ratings of the safety climate.

The 2009 study added qualitative data to the 2003 results and has helped in getting physicians on board, notes Suzanne Graham, RN, PhD, director of patient safety for KP's California regions.

Focus on safe care

The goal of Highly Reliable Surgical Teams is to "create teamwork, engagement, and a culture of safety where everyone is focused on giving safe care," says Laura Moreno, RN, BSN, MBA, clinical practice leader for patient safety for KP's Northern California region.

Some characteristics are:
- open communication
- a flattened hierarchy in the OR
- standardizing processes like the time-out and briefings
- becoming a "learning organization"—an organization that enables learning and continuously improves
- adopting best practices.

Five traits of high reliability organizations

Sensitivity to operations
Leaders and staff have constant awareness of the state of systems and processes that affect patient care. This awareness is key to noticing risks and preventing them.

Reluctance to simplify
Simple processes are good. But simplistic explanations of why things work or fail are risky. Avoiding overly simple explanations—unqualified staff, inadequate training, communication failure, etc—is essential to understand the true reasons patients are placed at risk.

Preoccupation with failure
Near misses are viewed as evidence of systems that should be improved to reduce potential harm to patients.

Deference to expertise
Leaders and supervisors listen and respond to insights of staff who know how processes really work and the risks patients really face.

Resilience
Leaders and staff are trained and prepared to know how to respond when system failures do occur.

Source: Agency for Healthcare Research and Quality. Becoming a High Reliability Organization. www.ahrq.gov/qual/hroadvice/hroadviceexecsum.htm

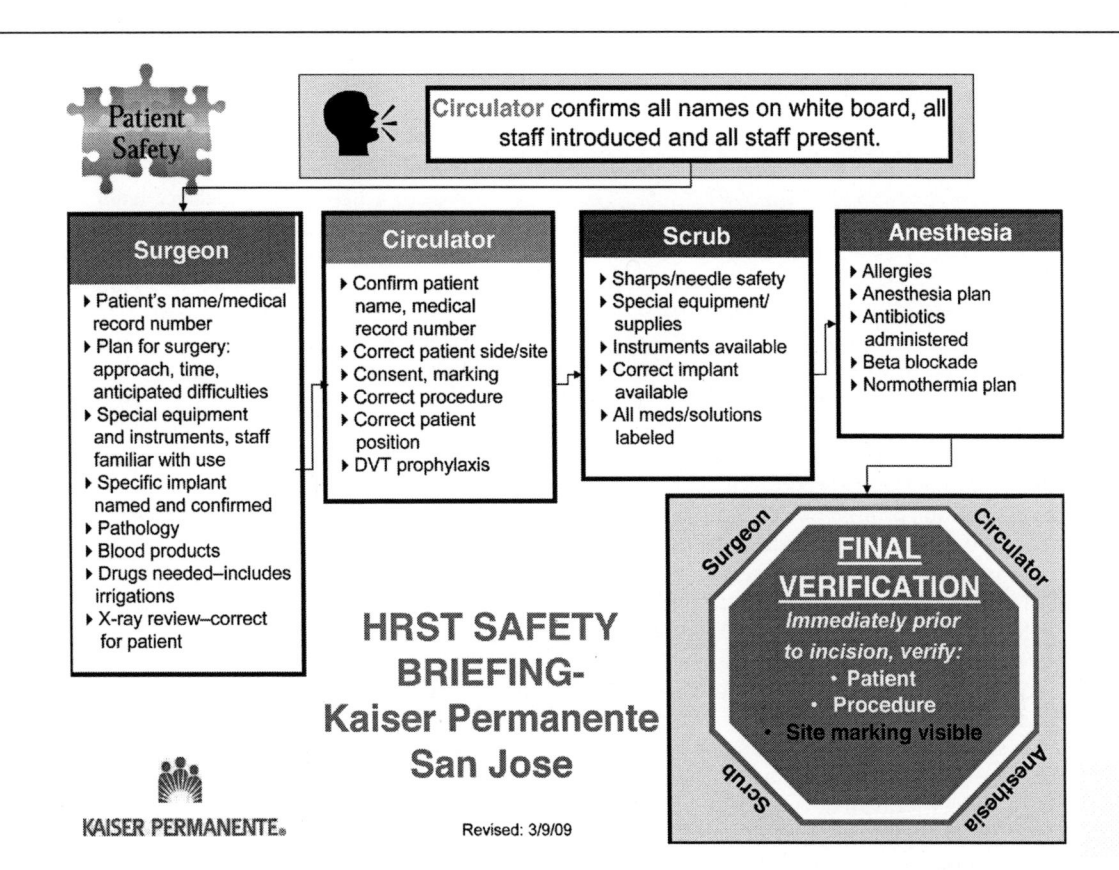

HRST SAFETY BRIEFING- Kaiser Permanente San Jose

Patient Safety

Circulator confirms all names on white board, all staff introduced and all staff present.

Surgeon
- Patient's name/medical record number
- Plan for surgery: approach, time, anticipated difficulties
- Special equipment and instruments, staff familiar with use
- Specific implant named and confirmed
- Pathology
- Blood products
- Drugs needed—includes irrigations
- X-ray review—correct for patient

Circulator
- Confirm patient name, medical record number
- Correct patient side/site
- Consent, marking
- Correct procedure
- Correct patient position
- DVT prophylaxis

Scrub
- Sharps/needle safety
- Special equipment/supplies
- Instruments available
- Correct implant available
- All meds/solutions labeled

Anesthesia
- Allergies
- Anesthesia plan
- Antibiotics administered
- Beta blockade
- Normothermia plan

FINAL VERIFICATION
Immediately prior to incision, verify:
- Patient
- Procedure
- Site marking visible

(Surgeon, Circulator, Scrub, Anesthesia)

KAISER PERMANENTE. Revised: 3/9/09

Expert teams

For the 19 KP Northern California medical centers, the high reliability effort is guided by an expert team of physician and nurse leaders. In developing the program, they studied the literature and KP's own data, including root causes of sentinel events, and found, not surprisingly, common themes were teamwork and communication.

The experts began meeting with representatives from the medical centers and asked, "What does the ideal OR look like?" They developed surgical safety tools, such as a preop briefing script and piloted the tools in 3 medical centers.

The project was rolled out to all 21 facilities in 2007 and 2008. Each medical center was asked to:

- identify a Highly Reliable Surgical Team leadership group with a surgeon champion, OR manager or director, and quality representative
- conduct human-factors and critical-event training
- administer the Safety Attitudes Questionnaire (SAQ) to measure how physicians, nurses, and support staff currently feel about issues such as teamwork, communication, and perceptions of management
- develop a standardized template for preoperative briefings
- begin performing consistent briefings in every OR for every case.

Visual aid for briefings

As an aid to briefings, KP's San Jose Medical Center came up with a visual tool that can be used as a poster or a laminated sheet on a clip board (illustration).

"They put the poster up in the OR so everyone understands the roles and the script," Moreno says.

KP teams are asked to do the briefing before anesthesia induction with the patient in the OR, which raised some eyebrows at first, she notes. There are exceptions, such as pediatric cases.

"Everyone comes together before induction," she explains. "The patient is awake. They introduce themselves and start the briefing.

"We have made it a hard stop," she adds, "and the staff and surgeons will not hand over the knife until the briefing is completed."

Despite some hesitation about patients hearing the briefing, teams have found patients actually find it reassuring. Some patients even join in, volunteering their name and the procedure to be done.

The tipping point

To reach the tipping point where a highly reliable culture is a way of life, Graham says support by 3 parties is critical—senior leadership, surgeon champions, and perioperative directors and managers.

"Our top surgical leader for Northern California is a staunch backer in supporting culture change," Graham says. At the facility level, surgeon champions have intervened when peers have resisted briefings and other safety strategies.

Study of teamwork behaviors

The Kaiser Permanente study involved RN observations of 300 surgical procedures and an assessment of 30-day postoperative outcomes.

Observers rated each surgical team from 0 to 4 based on team behaviors that have been shown to contribute to performance. Examples are briefing, information sharing, and assertion. The procedures were rated for low, medium, or high risk of complications. The 30-day outcome for each procedure was determined by medical record review.

Each procedure team was given a single behavior score. The researchers then calculated the relationship between the behavior score and the odds ratio for complications and death.

In findings, patients whose surgical teams showed less teamwork behaviors were at a higher risk for death or complications, even after adjusting for their risk category.

The authors say the results provide "general support for the development of team training for surgical teams."

Source: Mazzocco K, Petitti D B, Fong K T. Am J Surg. 2009;197: 678-685.

To aid the evolution, project leaders from the regional office visit the medical centers to conduct independent observations of briefings and offer feedback.

Scoring safety

The KP medical centers track their progress by keeping a "surgical safety dashboard" that includes:
- conduct of briefings
- compliance with metrics for the Surgical Care Improvement Project (SCIP), such as on-time administration of antibiotics and venous thromboembolism prevention
- any "never events" (events that should never happen to patients)
- SAQ scores for the safety culture and teamwork.

The briefings are scored on 3 elements:
- Leadership: Was the surgeon leading the briefing and actively engaged?
- Script: Was the script followed by each participant?
- Engagement: Was everyone attentive during the briefing?

"We set a benchmark that we want these to happen 90% of the time," Moreno says.

Over a year, the medical centers were able to bring their SCIP scores, which had varied, closer together and into the 90th percentile.

"We think the briefings were a key element in improving our SCIP scores," she notes.

The GLITCH list

KP medical centers are also encouraged to adopt debriefings at the end of surgical cases. The purpose is to discuss what went well and what could be improved.

Some centers are compiling information from the debriefings into what they call GLITCH lists—Gather Little Insights That Can Help. The lists include issues that need to be addressed, such as equipment problems or systems problems. The manager is responsible for seeing that GLITCH issues are followed up and addressed. The issues are reviewed monthly by the leadership team.

"The debriefings have really heightened communication between the staff and surgeons and helped to address some of the 'pebbles in their shoes,'" says Moreno. Equipment issues seem to be the most common topic.

"This really has been a collaborative effort that has brought together our departments of quality, patient care services, and the physicians," Moreno says. "They have been able to effect change by having this triad work together." ❖

References

Agency for Healthcare Research and Quality. Becoming a Highly Reliable Organization: Operational Advice for Hospital Leaders. April 2008. www.ahrq.gov/qual/hroadvice/

Leonard M, Graham S, Bonacum D. The human factor: The critical importance of effective teamwork and communication in providing safe care. *Qual Saf Health Care.* 2004;13(Suppl):i85-i90.

Mazzocco K, Petitti D B, Fong K T. Surgical team behaviors and patient outcomes. *Am J Surg.* 2009;197:678-685.

"Preflight checklist" builds safety culture, reduces nurse turnover. *OR Manager.* 2003;19(12):1, 8-10.

This article originally appeared in OR Manager, *February 2010;26:16-18.*

Team Agreement, Competition Boost Record for On-Time Starts

With health care reform looming and the financial picture for hospitals uncertain, perioperative leaders know senior executives will look to the OR as a major source of revenue. That's likely to increase pressure to improve OR performance. Starting cases on time in the morning is one way surgeons judge an OR's customer service and responsiveness.

For a Harrisburg, Pennsylvania-based health system, a team agreement and some friendly competition have helped improve on-time starts. PinnacleHealth launched the program in January 2010 after a year-long effort to collect data, streamline preoperative care, and forge a team agreement for on-time starts among the surgeons, anesthesia providers, and perioperative staff.

"We did not implement this until we felt we were a hundred percent ready in each area," says Susan Comp, RN, BSN, MS, CNOR, director of surgical services for Harrisburg-based PinnacleHealth, which has 2 campuses.

"Prior to this project, we did not see any urgency in getting patients prepared for surgery. Now I see that everyone is helping each other."

When the project began, only 13% of cases at the 19-OR Harrisburg Campus and 7% at the 9-OR Community Campus started on time.

Surgeons were unhappy. In a survey, they said overwhelmingly that it was very important to them to start on time.

By April 2010, 100% of ORs had started on time for 4 out of 5 days at Harrisburg and 3 out of 5 days at Community. In June, Comp said the ORs were still meeting 100% on most days.

On-time reports

"Our goal was for 90% of first-case patients to be wheeled into the OR on time. We never expected to achieve 100% as many times as we have," she says. The goal remains at 90% because some delays are inevitable.

"There are still reasons for late starts, such as patient issues. But the staff, anesthesia providers, or surgeon being late is no longer the number one reason we are not on time."

The help of a Six Sigma Black Belt, Cindy Wilson, RN, which PinnacleHealth provided, was instrumental, Comp says.

"The Six Sigma process is one of the best I've been involved in. You define, measure, analyze, improve, and control the entire project.

"We now have the data when we are questioned by a physician who says, 'I wasn't late those days.'"

Under the team agreement, physicians sign in when they arrive so the time is captured.

Wilson created an on-time report that is sent to the surgeons each week. After she moves on to other projects, an OR staff member will keep up the data collection and reporting.

These are major features of the program.

Team agreement on start time

A cornerstone of the project is a team agreement that spells out requirements as well as rewards and consequences for surgeons, anesthesia providers, and staff.

A key step was reaching consensus on the definition of an on-time start. Polling the staff and physicians, the project team found a consensus that 7:30 am should be the start time, with patients wheeled into the OR by 7:25 am. Other time elements were also set (sidebar).

In the survey, the surgeons said they thought the only way to achieve on-time starts was to have a penalty system. The consequences are outlined in the team agreement. Once consensus was reached, the formal team agreement was endorsed by the OR committee, which consists primarily of surgeons and serves as the OR's governing body. The senior administration also endorsed the project, so leaders knew they had support if a surgeon complained.

Large copies of the team agreement are posted throughout the department.

Improving the preop process

One factor in late starts was a preop process that needed a tuneup.

Gathering data, the project team found the time it took to prepare outpatients and same-day admissions "was all over the board," Comp says. Consulting with the staff, they learned there was no systematic way of assigning a nurse to a patient, and many RNs thought certain activities weren't their job.

"We came to the conclusion that it's everybody's job to take care of a patient," Comp says.

Steps were taken to streamline the process and define responsibilities for RNs and clinical assistants (sidebar, p 24).

Improving the preop process

These are steps taken by Pinnacle Health.

Barriers
- Time wasted at the desk and at the time of handoff.
- OR staff complaints about delays in completing paperwork.
- Inconsistent process by the staff.

First steps to improvement
- Timed 5 staff members for 10 same-day admits and short procedure patients.
- Watched the process and gathered data for 6 weeks.

Plan
- Set time frames for preop preparation:
  —55 minutes for same-day admit patients
  —35 minutes for short-procedure patients.

Prioritized daily tasks
- Bring patients into unit using visual cues from the patient tracking system.
- Standardize the chart process. Place charts that are ready in a designated rack.
- If a bay is empty, any available staff member (RN or clinical assistant) cleans it and brings in a stretcher and a patient.
- Begin the admission process.

Before patient assessment
- Review chart only for information needed, not the whole chart.
- Gather supplies.

At the bedside
- Begin perioperative charting.
- Look up lab test results.

Followup
- Provide patient education.
- Finalize preoperative checklist and prepare patient for surgery.

"One thing we struggle with is time management," Comp says. Some staff knew while others needed more guidance.

Now completed patient charts are placed in a file. Nurses take the first chart from the file and begin caring for the patient. Previously, nurses went through the file to select the patient they wanted to take care of.

Leaders are setting up productivity measures for the number of admissions a day an RN is expected to complete.

Rewards and consequences

A voluntary reward system has been a surprise hit with surgeons and staff, injecting a bit of fun. Rewards are spelled out on cards personnel carry in their badge holders. Being on time earns a star sticker. Anyone who earns 15 stars is eligible for a small prize, such as a pen. The maximum number of stars is 50, which earns a jacket embroidered with the winner's name.

"I've never seen surgeons so excited," Comp says. "They push each other to earn the stars."

There are also consequences, spelled out in the team agreement. Surgeons who are late 3 times in a quarter are at risk to lose one morning block for a month.

A surgeon is documented as late when the patient is unable to be taken to the OR at 7:20 am because the surgeon arrived after 7:15 am and was not finished with the patient in time for the patient to arrive in the OR by 7:25 am.

Data for surgeons with 3 late arrivals is sent to the OR committee for review. Surgeons may submit an appeal form, which is reviewed by the committee before reaching a decision about the penalty. If a surgeon to be penalized is part of a group that has a block, the group will lose access to the block time for a month.

Consequences for anesthesiologists and staff are governed by hospital policies.

Though some physicians objected to the penalties, Comp says administrators backed the decision, and a few surgeons lost block time.

"It only takes one physician to lose a block to make everyone think, 'Wow, they're serious,'" she says, adding that nearly all surgeons are on time.

"The surgeons who are on time every day are happy, and they have been supporting this," she says.

"Our managers have also been excellent. They have taken a lot of heat and stood their ground. This has been more successful than we ever thought it would be."

Lessons learned

Comp offered this advice for other OR teams addressing on-time starts:
- Take the time, 6 months or even a year, to evaluate your process to understand the barriers to starting on time.

"We wanted to move forward quicker, but we knew that if we didn't fix our process before we started, we would not be successful," Comp says.

- Make sure the project has senior leadership support.

- Involve the physicians from the beginning. Seek agreement on the on-time start initiative from the OR's governing body, including representatives of each surgical specialty.
- Communicate often. "Everyone was tired of seeing letters in the mail and posters in the lounges. Still, there were a few who said they didn't know about it," she says.

The program was pilot-tested in January 2010 and fully rolled out in February. In June, the team planned to start the next project—on-time starts for 12:30 pm cases. ❖

This article originally appeared in OR Manager, *August 2010;26:1,8-10.*

Data Sparks On-Time Improvements

As with most busy ORs, we were looking to improve our efficiency. Consultants were brought in and gave recommendations, but it did not change our culture or improve our on-time starts. We had meetings with anesthesia providers, surgeons, and nurses. The results were differing opinions on the definition of an "on-time start," the lack of credibility of the data, who determined the cause of the delay, potential bias, and lack of accountability.

As someone who has heard many of these conversations over the years, I wanted to make a change. I wanted to provide accurate data that reflected the true causes of our delays.

As a pediatric tertiary referral center and Level I trauma center with 12 staffed ORs, we perform complex surgery, including open-heart procedures, cranial reconstructions, and posterior spinal fusions. Our patients may have several co-morbidities, with more than one service involved in their care. These factors contribute to complicated setups and multidisciplinary coordination, which also affects first case on-time starts.

Involving nursing staff

I knew the nursing staff would be integral in offering insight, providing suggestions and helping to influence change.

I had several conversations with the nursing staff, explaining that the purpose of collecting data was to identify areas for improvement. I wanted to ensure they understood there were not negative consequences for them if nursing was the cause of the delay. The intent was to help them to get first-case patients into the ORs on time by providing the support they needed.

Collecting data

In January 2009, I started manually collecting data on a daily basis. I reviewed the charts of each patient who had a first-case start, documenting the date, surgeon, anesthesiologist, time scheduled, time in room, cause of delay, and nursing/technologist staff in the room. The causes of delays are documented in the perioperative nursing information system.

The average first-case on-time start for January 2009 was 21%, meaning the patient arrived in the OR room on time. In February 2009, 22% of first cases were in the OR room on time. (Previously, we had reached consensus that a case would be considered late if the patient arrived into the OR more than 5 minutes past the scheduled in-room time.)

Data starts discussions

The percentage of on-time starts was posted daily on the add-on board at the front of the department. Posting the on-time starts generated discussion and brought the data to everyone's attention.

I continued to have conversations with the nursing staff and started to meet with the chief of anesthesia and chief of surgery. I asked that we set aside differences and blame and trust each other. We had to have a starting point and take action on what we could improve.

After I had collected a few months of data, trends became evident. I met with the chief of anesthesia and reviewed the data I had collected. He started having discussions with his group, which is contracted with the hospital.

I also met with the chief of surgery and reviewed the data. He asked for a separate report that showed delays by individual surgeon. He followed up with individual surgeons, often that same day, and helped to bring awareness to unnecessary delays. He also asked that each surgeon receive a copy of his or her individual delay data. Our CEO and the department chairs helped provide leadership in setting expectations.

As the months passed, and the data spoke for itself, it helped to reinforce that we were on the right track. Throughout the year, data was presented to the nursing staff and the OR committee. This enabled everyone to see the progress being made. It also offered an opportunity to hear feedback and suggestions for improvement.

Results show improvement

From January through December 2009, we improved on-time starts from 21% to a 60% high, with an average of 47.25% for the year. Comparing the first quarter of 2009 (25%) to the first quarter of 2010 (62%), we have improved by 37%. I am also very proud to say we have had several days that 100% of first cases started on time.

Nursing makes changes

As we collected the data and our on-time starts improved, we realized nursing would need to make some changes. Issues were discussed at staff meetings and during rounds. We brainstormed for ideas and solutions that would help and implemented the following:

- A third staff member was added to the night shift so there would be adequate staff to manage first cases and prepare the rooms.
- Staffing in the postanesthesia care unit was adjusted to have nurses arrive earlier for the number of ORs finishing at 8 am to 8:30 am.
- First-case patients and same-day surgery staff were scheduled to arrive one-half hour earlier because, with surgeons and anesthesia providers arriving earlier, nurses had less time with patients.
- Having patients ready on time placed more pressure on the OR nurses to prepare rooms for complex cases. Nurses have used that time but feel rushed and stressed to get into the room on time. We are having discussions on how to improve this situation, which includes providing a second circulator for complex cases, having night shift staff assist the circulator with opening supplies, confirming implants with sterile processing the night before, checking on blood, and possibly providing more ancillary support.

We have also discussed having OR staff arrive earlier or changing our expectation for OR nurses to be in the room by 7 am instead of 7:10 am. Through all the discussions, we have reinforced that the goal is to provide what is needed to help nurses bring patients to the OR safely and on time.

A special challenge

Our craniofacial patients often require a multidisciplinary team and present a challenge in getting them prepared on the morning of surgery. To allow for preop preparation, we would like these patients to be seen in the preop clinic the day before surgery, but many families cannot afford the extra expense of a hotel. We are exploring possible housing options and financial assistance for these patients and families so any issues can be addressed and resolved the day before instead of causing a delay on the morning of surgery.

On-time incentives

At this point, our incentives involve giving a lot of positive feedback on improvements and recognizing those efforts. Regarding penalties, surgeons have been notified recently that if they are consistently late, their 7:30 am start time will be given to another surgeon.

Advice for other managers

My advice for other managers is to start with accurate data collection and to post the percentage of on-time starts. I did not have any formal meetings or discussions with physicians.

In retrospect, I would have had even more conversations with nursing staff on all shifts to explain the goal and intent of the data collection. Some physicians expect the charge nurses to have an immediate fix or hold them accountable for any delay problem.

Examples of delays

Surgeon: 58
Late: 26
No consent: 21
Working elsewhere: 11

Anesthesia: 23
Consent: 14
Anesthesia late: 5
Talk with family: 2
Needed in another OR: 1
Complex setup: 1
(Anesthesia equipment: 6)

Patient/family: 43
Had questions: 30
Late: 9
Speak with doctor: 4

Preop medication/ testing: 16

OR: 13
Complex setup: 11
Change in assignments: 2

Transport: 18
Inpatient unit not ready: 11
Delay: 7

The staff nurses can be caught in the middle between anesthesia providers and surgeons because they are documenting the reason for the delay. The nursing staff has to know they are supported, and there will be followup if they are verbally harassed or feel patient care is compromised.

Data generate discussion and interest. Review the data with anyone who will listen and gain support from physician leadership. Be prepared for questions and pushback, because some individuals will be defensive, and some will not want to change.

When facing resistance, I suggested that we could continue to rehash the same conversations we have had for years, or we could all make a choice to take action and make improvements. I also reinforce that it takes the whole team working together to be successful in improving on-time starts. ❖

—LeAnn Northam, RN, MSN, CNOR
Clinical Manager,
Riley Operating Room
Riley Hospital for Children
Indianapolis

Benchmarking the OR's Key Indicators

Surgeons at St Vincent's Hospital in Bridgeport, Connecticut, were frustrated because the scheduled start times for their cases during the day seemed to vary a lot.

Using their new dashboard, OR leaders were able to see that they were below the benchmark for scheduling accuracy.

"We were not doing a good job with accurately posting the case durations," says Brooke Karlsen, BSN, MSN, RN, the director of surgical services.

To address the situation, she and her colleagues are starting a project to measure setup and cleanup times for the top 10 surgeons and their top 10 procedures. "We think we have underestimated those numbers and have made some adjustments," she says.

St Vincent's Surgery Dashboard

Indicator	Actual	Peer Group Mean	Achievement against Benchmark
% First Case On-Time or Early ± 5	71.7%	54.8%	130.84% ✓
% Subsequent Case On-Time or Early	26.2%	42.8%	61.21% ✗
Patient In to Patient Out (min)	115.7	144.0	124.46% ✓
Patient In to Anesthesia Ready (min)	16.6	14.0	84.34% ✗
Patient In to Incision (min)	16.7	34.0	203.59% ✓
Incision to Close (min)	88.4	97.0	109.73% ✓
Close to Patient Out (min)	10.7	12.0	112.15% ✓
Average Turnover Minutes (min)	31.9	33.0	103.45% ✓
% Scheduling Accuracy	35.1%	32.4%	108.33% ✓
% Utilized 7am-3pm	69%	77.2%	89.38% ✗
% Utilized 3pm-5pm	60%	75.5%	79.47% ✗
% Utilized 5pm-7pm	48%	68.4%	70.18% ✗
% Utilized 7pm-11pm	10%	65.5%	15.27% ✗
% Same Day Add-On	3.8%	14.6%	384.21% ✓
% Block Utilization	68.4%	65.0%	105.23% ✓
% of Schedule Blocked	25.2%	‡	+
% Same Day Cancelled/Postponed	4.6%	15.8%	343.48% ✓
% Patients Screened Prior to Surgery	‡	58.7%	+
% Surgical Checklist/Timeout Compliance	100.0%	98.5%	101.52% ✓
% Returns to Surgery within 24 hrs	0.1%	‡	+

Legend
✓ Measure meets or exceeds target
✗ Measure does not meet target
‡ Information unavailable
+ Achievement cannot be calculated

Karlsen, with the chief of surgery, Douglas Ross, MD, who joined the organization 2 years ago, have been on a mission to create a more data-driven OR. The hospital recently subscribed to the OR Benchmarks Collaborative (ORBC), a collaboration between OR Manager, Inc, and McKesson.

"We worked with ORBC to create a custom dashboard based on the corporate goals for our hospital," Karlsen says. Metrics include:
- main OR first case on-time starts
- main OR turnover time
- total joint volume
- ambulatory surgery first case on-time starts
- ambulatory surgery turnover time
- same-day canceled cases
- first-case start delays caused by improperly prepared case carts
- subsequent-case delays caused by improperly prepared case carts.

The OR had made some progress before, such as bringing its first-case on-time start percentages from the teens to the 70s. But these efforts required custom reports developed by its IT specialist.

"We really didn't have a way to benchmark how we compare with others," Karlsen says.

With ORBC's web-based service, St Vincent's submits its data monthly and then can access an online scorecard and dashboard showing how the OR is doing on key performance indicators. The scorecard can be used to drill down for more detail, identify causes of poor performance, and create custom reports.

For some metrics, it's going to be a stretch, Karlsen acknowledges. "On others, we were kind of surprised—we were doing better than we thought." Same-day case cancellations and block time utilization, for example, were at or above the 90th percentile for the benchmark.

Dashboard summary

Audience: OR leadership team (chief of surgery, director of surgical services, chief of anesthesia, managers, assistant nurse manager, OR scheduling manager, sterile processing manager, educator); staff; and physicians.

Metrics: OR operational performance indicators.

Frequency: Monthly.

Software: The dashboard is created using ORBC's vendor-neutral business intelligence software. St Vincent's uses McKesson's PerSe OR information system. ❖

This article originally appeared in OR Manager, *February 2011;27:12-13.*

Handoffs: What ORs Can Learn From Formula One Race Crews

Hospitals are taking lessons from the high performance of Formula 1 racing pit-stop crews and applying them to handoffs between the OR and the ICU.

"The handoff is like a pit stop: surgery is the first section of the race, the second part is intensive care, and the handoff is in the middle," says Ken Catchpole, PhD, senior postdoctoral scientist in the Quality, Reliability, Safety and Teamwork Unit at the Nuffield Department of Surgical Sciences at the University of Oxford in England.

"You have to do lots of different things under time pressure, and if you make a mistake, it can have consequences down the road." In a race, for example, a wheel not tightened correctly can fall off and cause an accident.

Catchpole worked with 2 physicians who were inspired by watching pit-stop crews in action on television to explore what lessons could be applied to handoffs between surgery and the ICU. Pit-stop crews excel at what they do: It takes them only about 7 seconds to change tires and refuel the car and, more importantly, no driver has died behind the wheel since 1994.

"What they were doing was incredibly reliable, but what we were doing in health care was far less reliable," says Catchpole, who points out that all safety efforts involve people. "People working in health care and in racing are all human, and humans make similar mistakes."

Based on conversations and videotaping, Catchpole's team created a new transfer protocol for the Great Ormond Street Hospital (GOSH) for Children in London. The change paid off. A study in *Pediatric Anesthesia* in 2007 found that implementing the new handoff protocol significantly reduced the number of omissions of information and technical errors in patients transferred from the OR to the ICU.

Spreading the word

Other countries, including the US, have adapted the GOSH model. The University of California San Francisco Medical Center (UCSF) has been using the model for about a year, according to Marilyn Irovando, RN, patient manager of the pediatric cardiac ICU and pediatric interventional cardiology.

"Root cause analysis showed us errors occurred because the postop plan wasn't known to everyone." she says. "The new protocol has all members integral to the transfer and receipt of information present at the point of patient transfer from OR to ICU care." The team, which includes either the primary surgeon or his designee, the anesthesiologist, the medical ICU attending physician, and the primary receiving RN, then discuss management strategies for the next 12 to 24 hours.

At Children's Hospital Boston, Patricia Hickey, PhD, MBA, RN, FAAN, VP of cardiac and critical care services, says the GOSH model has helped "break down the traditional barriers between disciplines." Previously, the OR nurse and anesthesiologist "would give separate reports, which caused gaps and people hearing the information differently," she says. "Now the entire team (surgeon, anesthesiologist, and OR and ICU nurses) is present so questions are answered in real time."

Lessons from behind the wheel

Research published in *Quality and Safety in Health Care* reports health care professionals can learn 3 primary lessons from Formula 1 teams:
- proactive learning with briefings and checklists to prevent errors
- active management using technology to transfer information
- posthoc learning from the storage and analysis of electronic data records.

Catchpole adds, "Processes help a team work better. Even if you have a less effective team but an effective process, you will do relatively well. Of course, you want to have both."

An effective team communicates well and anticipates problems. In addition to teamwork, it's important to have leadership training, identify task sequences, and implement checklists.

Before making any change, however, Irovando says, "You need to gain consensus that a change is necessary, that it facilitates patient safety, and that it won't negatively impact workflow."

As with most change, a multidisciplinary approach is key, says Hickey. The new model was discussed at the ICU practice committee meeting, and the OR manager sat on the subcommittee that formalized the plan.

Catchpole says developing an effective handoff protocol includes reducing variability, identifying tasks and assigning responsibility, providing education and an easy-to-use resource, and measuring results.

Example: OR-to-ICU transfer

Purpose

To improve continuity of patient care through effective communication during transition from the cardiovascular OR (CVOR) to the cardiac ICU (CICU).

Procedure

Prior to patient transfer
- CVOR nurse will complete the Nurse-to-Nurse Report Form and give verbal telephone report to the CICU nurse accepting the patient transfer.
- CVOR nurse, cardiac anesthesia attending and fellow, and cardiac surgery fellow will transport the patient to the CICU.

On arrival to the CICU
- CICU nurse will connect patient to monitors.
- CICU attending and fellow, respiratory therapist, and charge nurse will be paged to the patient bedside.
- Once the patient has been connected to the monitors, the cardiac anesthesia attending is satisfied the patient is in stable condition, and all clinical disciplines are represented, a structured sign-out will occur in the following order:
  — Anesthesia fellow or attending will describe pre-bypass management of the patient including pre-operative medication, induction of anesthesia, airway management, and events.
  — Cardiac surgery fellow or attending will describe the surgical findings and repair including assessment of repair, potential concerns and complications, transesophageal echo findings, and hemodynamic data.
  — Cardiac anesthesia attending/fellow will describe the post-bypass course including hemodynamic stability and support, ventilatory management, and any additional concerns such as dysrhythmias or bleeding.
  — CVOR nurse will describe any additional patient or family concerns and confirm the last dose of antibiotics and blood product availability.
  — The CICU attending or fellow will provide a feedback summary of report and discuss the plan for patient care to close the communication loop.

Courtesy of Children's Hospital Boston.

Reducing variability

"Every cardiac surgery patient is different, but the care each receives should be similar," he says. "It's important to know why differences occur so variability can be reduced." He compares it to purchasing a car—the buyer can specify different items, such as the color or number of doors, but the car is still the same brand.

That doesn't mean variations are eliminated. "You need to know when you are deviating from the standard and make that decision consciously," says Catchpole. For example, a patient with several comorbid diseases may require more intensive care than one with one primary problem.

To reduce variability, Children's Hospital Boston, uses a form that outlines the specifics of what is needed in the handoff report. "There isn't a set structure," says Patti Galvin, MSN, RN, CNOR, manager of the cardiac OR. "All the elements of patient care are listed, and each discipline goes through its part. It breaks down the silos."

The anesthesiologist covers topics such as the anesthesia induction and any arrhythmias or blood pressure problems, while the surgeon reports on the surgical procedure that was done.

"The OR nurse covers any piece that's left out," says Galvin. That might include antibiotics, blood products, or family concerns. The ICU team documents what was said and reads it back to verify it is correct.

UCSF's OR-to-ICU handoff protocol states that the surgeon reports on the surgical procedure and significant intraoperative events, and the ICU nurse follows specific instructions such as minimizing nonessential bedside conversation and holding blood draws until after report. The anesthesiologist gives a detailed report on specifics, ranging from the patient's preoperative history to intraoperative medication administration. Questions from the bedside RN and the ICU fellow and attending physician are included as part of the process.

Identifying tasks and assigning responsibility

Developing the GOSH model meant each handoff task had to be identified, says Catchpole. "We looked at what is required for each task, who should be doing it, and when it should happen in the process." He notes that like pit-stop crews who break down tasks into individual movements, such as taking the wheel off and putting it back on, clinicians need to delve into that level of detail.

Identifying task sequences can be particularly helpful. "We found the patient would come in (to the ICU), and everyone would be busy connecting the monitors, so no one was listening to the doctor giving report," says Catchpole. The new protocol delayed the verbal report until the patient was placed on the monitors.

"Everyone has an individual job in a pit-stop crew," Catchpole notes. This helps avoid confusion and task omission. Before the new protocol, "No one was sure who should do what, and some tasks, like plugging in the infusion pump, had 2 people." When 2 people are responsible, each might think the other is doing the task, resulting in a task left undone.

The 'lollipop man'

A key leadership role is similar to the "lollipop man," the person at the pit stop who makes the decision whether to delay the car going back on the track. "That job is critical," says Catchpole. "They don't physically do anything, but they are the most important member of the team." At GOSH, the lollipop man in the OR/ICU handoff is the surgeon.

At Children's Hospital Boston, an OR nurse accompanies the patient to the ICU to give report. "Another nurse starts the next case so we don't hold up the OR schedule," says Galvin. In the ICU, 2 nurses, the charge nurse, and the surgeon admit the patient.

Providing education and resources

Staff and surgeons need to learn about the new handoff process along with other communication tools. Simulation can help accomplish those goals.

"We have used simulation for team training and communication," says Galvin. "One of the (simulation) cases is transferring a patient to the CVOR."

The entire OR team, including nurses, surgical and perfusion technologists, surgeons, and anesthesiologists, completes simulation training twice a year.

Catchpole recommends having a clinician-oriented resource that goes through the entire process. "Then we added a checklist to fill in the critical information that is needed," he says. "If the nurse wasn't told a piece of expected information, such as how long cross-clamping occurred, she would be prompted to ask."

Catchpole cautions that checklists can "make more work." To avoid that problem, at GOSH, the checklist is the admission entry for the patient, so nurses don't have to reenter information.

Measuring results

Measuring results not only helps demonstrate what is working but also demonstrates to staff the value of the change.

"It was apparent that the new protocol was easier to do instead of the way they had been doing it," says Catchpole.

Of course, adaptation is key for the entire process. "What we did worked for us," says Catchpole. "People might take those ideas and use them in different ways."

Crossing the finish line

"About 50% of process improvement is not what you do but how you go about it," says Catchpole. "We took time to get the experts involved to learn the right lessons and to talk through what we were learning with the people who were doing the work. It's about how you work with other professionals to change the way they work."

"What it comes down to is that we need to understand how to help people perform better," he adds.

Using a pit stop analogy "brings everyone together and makes the patient the center of the activity," says Galvin. "It is an exemplar for a healthy work environment." ❖

—*Cynthia Saver, MS, RN*

Cynthia Saver is a freelance writer in Columbia, Maryland.

References

Catchpole K, Sellers R, Goldman A, et al. Patient handovers within the hospital: translating knowledge from motor racing to healthcare. *Qual Saf Health Care*. 2010;19:318-322.

Catchpole K R, de Leval M R, McEwan A, et al. Patient handover from surgery to intensive care: using Formula 1 pit-stop and aviation models to improve safety and quality. *Paediatr Anaesth*. 2007;17:470-478.

This article originally appeared in OR Manager, *April 2011;27:1,11-13.*

Looking to Front-Line Clinicians, Staff for Lasting Improvements

A patient with a multidrug-resistant infection is coming to your OR. That patient will travel from her room—one of the most contaminated areas of the hospital—to surgery, which is perhaps the cleanest. How can her caregivers avoid cross-contamination that could transmit the infection to others?

At 219-bed St Patrick Hospital and Health Sciences Center in Missoula, Montana, the answer is to look to its front-line clinicians and staff as well as for best practices from outside the organization. The approach, called Positive Deviance, or PD, stems from the idea that the best and most lasting improvements come from clinicians and staff who care for patients every day.

"Positive Deviance is based on the premise that solutions to tough problems that have not responded to traditional approaches already exist within the community that faces the problem," explains Jon Lloyd, MD, a surgeon and a proponent of PD. He is coaching hospitals on PD projects centered on eliminating transmission of Methicillin-resistant *Staphylococcus aureus* (MRSA) (sidebar).

"PD enables the community to discover and spread its own hidden solutions so everybody has access to them and the opportunity to adopt the same successful behaviors and strategies," he says.

How PD works

One question St Patrick wanted to address was: How do we transport patients infected or colonized with multidrug-resistant organisms (MDRO) so the receiving unit, such as the OR, understands that these patients require special precautions? And what does the receiving unit need to do to prevent transmission while these patients are being cared for on that unit? (MRSA and *Clostridium difficile* were 2 MDROs of concern.)

Professional guidelines for preventing MDRO transmission don't directly address the details of patient transfer.

In getting started with PD, Dr Lloyd explains, the first step is to involve senior administrators and clinical leaders so they understand how PD works and how results are measured. Then there is an invitation to opt in or opt out.

"PD engages only those people who want to use this approach to solve a problem," he notes.

If senior leaders opt in, they are invited to bring their employees together for a kickoff to explain PD and how it might work at the hospital.

Hospital employees can opt in or opt out. Those who opt in are given opportunities to become actively engaged, for example, by organizing the initiative, being trained to facilitate the process, or determining performance parameters they want to follow to track performance.

"Only those who are passionate to be involved in preventing health care-acquired infections (HAIs) are involved—it's all voluntary," Dr Lloyd says. "No one is assigned, designated, or appointed to be involved. Over time, word gets around, and more people get involved."

No consultants are involved. "It doesn't work if outside experts come in to facilitate the process," he adds. "For tough problems that require behavior change, the real experts are the front-line staff."

A core group meets to organize how to apply PD to a problem.

"It's best to start small and go slow so you can go fast," Dr Lloyd notes. Usually, hospitals start with one unit to build experience and make the case.

Introducing PD

St Patrick's employees were introduced to PD during the annual professional enrichment event, called APE. In small groups, they discussed what they do to prevent infections along with barriers and possible solutions, and reported back to the large group.

"In the first couple of APE sessions, a lot of OR people listed their barriers and frustrations" about patient transfers, notes Tammy Powers, BSN, RN, CIC, the infection prevention coordinator and a PD facilitator.

Powers saw this as an opportunity to create a core group of volunteers from day surgery, the hospital's 11 ORs, and the postanesthesia care unit (PACU) and hold "discovery and action dialogs," a PD technique for listening and drawing out ideas. In the core group were Powers; Carla Davies, BSN, RN, CNOR, OR manager; Michelle Sage, RN, CNOR, charge nurse; Michelle Leiby, BSN, RN, CPAN; and Ginger Martin RN, CMSRN.

What is Positive Deviance?

Positive Deviance is based on the observation that every community has certain individuals or groups whose uncommon behaviors and strategies enable them to find better solutions to problems than their peers, even though they have access to the same resources and face similar or worse challenges.

The Positive Deviance approach enables the community to discover these successful behaviors and strategies and develop a plan to promote their adoption.

Positive Deviance has been used to address issues such as child malnutrition, neonatal mortality, school drop-out, female genital cutting, hospital-acquired infections, and HIV/AIDS.

—*www.positivedeviance.org*

Who are the 'positive deviants'?

Front-line workers assess how the current process works. The facilitator acts as a catalyst who asks questions, not an expert with solutions. Then the core group identifies 'positive deviants'—those who do things differently or have ideas about how to improve the process.

Along with PD, the group decided to perform an A3, a Lean problem-solving process, for patient transfers. The team met 5 or 6 times and drew on other PD techniques, including skits and improvs, to work out a better process for patient transfer to and from the OR.

Solutions for patient transfers

These are some solutions for patient transfers that "positive deviants" identified. All solutions came from front-line staff such as RNs, nursing assistants, environmental services workers, patient transporters, and physicians.

Communication plan

Because communication was identified as a barrier, a communication plan for patient transfers was developed. The night before surgery, the charge nurse reviews the next day's schedule for patients who are flagged for an MDRO. Cases are flagged on the schedule, and "MDRO" is written on the time-out white board in the patient's OR as a reminder.

Transfer process

To refine the transport process:
- Patients positive for an MDRO are not transported to the OR in their own bed if at all possible. A clean stretcher is used instead.
- The patient is transported in a clean gown with clean hands and on clean linen. Depending on the surgery, a patient may have a preop shower or bath with chlorhexidine gluconate.
- Personal protective equipment (PPE) is worn in the patient's room. After the patient is on the stretcher and ready to be moved, the transporter cleans the side rails and head of the stretcher, removes the PPE, and performs hand hygiene. One "positive deviant" shared her idea to place the patient's chart in a belonging bag and hang it on the IV pole along with an isolation sign. This visual cue allows all personnel to recognize the need for contact precautions.
- If the patient must be transported in the bed, the bed is cleaned as well as possible.
- After the patient is transferred to the OR table, the stretcher is cleaned and placed back in service.
- Back in the patient's room, an environmental services worker cleans the patient's bed and changes the linens. The bed is then brought down to the OR to receive the patient after surgery, avoiding the need for multiple transfers after surgery.
- In the PACU, MDRO patients are placed in an isolation room.
- During surgery on MDRO patients, a runner is assigned, when available, to get supplies so the circulator won't have to make trips out of the OR to the supply core.

Anesthesia cart solution

An anesthesiologist offered ideas for better management of the anesthesia cart.

A special cart, identified by a red "racing stripe," was proposed for use in MDRO cases. The anesthesiologist suggested paring down the cart to essential supplies, with a fully stocked anesthesia cart outside the room.

The other anesthesiologists adopted the idea more readily than if it had come from outside their group, Powers notes.

Another innovation is to use plastic sandwich bags for storing small supplies such as needles and syringes in the cart. That way, an anesthesiologist can grab 3 bags of syringes and avoid potential contamination of syringes not needed for the case.

"When they go into the drawer and touch things, the surface of the bags can be wiped off," Davies explains. All of the anesthesia providers now use that method.

On board with PPE

Other ideas helped to determine how protective equipment (PPE) would be worn during patient transfers in the OR.

Guidelines of the Healthcare Infection Control Practices Advisory Committee (HICPAC) recommend that health care workers caring for patients on contact precautions wear a gown and gloves for all interactions that may involve contact with the patient or potentially contaminated areas of the patient's environment. The PPE is donned before or upon entering the room and discarded before exiting.

Using positive deviance to drive change in the OR

Positive Deviance has led to dramatic improvements in tough problems around the world, from improving the survival of low birth-weight babies in India, reducing school drop-out rates in California, or improving hand hygiene in hospitals.

In a general session at the 2011 Managing Today's OR Suite Conference, Jon C. Lloyd, MD, a surgeon and PD leader, talked about how ORs can use PD to lead change in their departments.

Dr Lloyd, a senior associate with the Positive Deviance Initiative at Tufts University, Boston, has coordinated an effort to eliminate endemic Methicillin-resistant *Staphylococcus aureus* in Veterans Affairs (VA) hospitals. A PD project in 2 Veterans Affairs hospitals in Pittsburgh started in 2005 led to a 50% reduction in MRSA infections, which was sustained and improved through 2009. The project included employee-generated ideas as well as established infection control protocols. (www.innovations.ahrq.gov/content.aspx?id=1853).

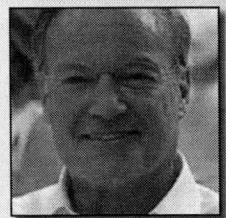

Jon C. Lloyd, MD

The results inspired and informed a 76% reduction in health care-associated MRSA infections in 153 VA hospital critical care units nationally.

Five non-VA hospitals have replicated the dramatic reductions in health care-associated-MRSA infections achieved by the Pittsburgh VA system, Dr Lloyd says. This effort was supported by the Centers for Disease Control and Prevention and the Robert Wood Johnson Foundation.

Learn more about PD at www.positivedeviance.org and www.plexusinstitute.org.

When an MDRO patient is brought into the OR, the entire team, including the circulating nurse and anesthesia provider, dons PPE while transferring the patient to the OR table. After the patient is draped, the anesthesia provider often continues to wear PPE, but the circulating nurse may remove PPE, discard it, and redon fresh PPE for transferring the patient to the PACU.

Once OR teams had a chance to observe and understand "what we were doing and why, we had much greater growth, especially with the anesthesia group," Davies says.

With use of PPE for MDRO cases, OR personnel are no longer required to change their scrub suits after the case.

"We now feel we can contain [the contamination] with PPE," she says.

Keeping PPE on hand

To make sure isolation gowns, gloves, MDRO signs, and cleaning supplies are handy, another "positive deviant" suggested a kit. Kits are placed on a table outside the OR where they are needed.

The day surgery unit has also developed a kit, and the OR offered them a spare cart to use. The cart also has a resource book and supplies such as disposable thermometers, blood pressure cuffs, and an isolation stethoscope.

"They got all of these supplies together in one afternoon, and it's been that way ever since," Powers notes.

Awareness about the need for contact precautions in the day surgery unit was raised when family members who had a patient with an MDRO on a medical unit started asking about wearing PPE when they were with the patient before and after surgery. The staff began making PPE available.

Environmental services management and staff have been involved from the beginning of the process.

"Our environmental services staff are very accommodating in helping us to reduce infections," Powers says.

What's different about PD?

How does positive deviance differ from other QI methods?

"PD helps you discover solutions you haven't tapped yet," Powers says. "If workers own the solutions and share them with their colleagues, the solutions are adopted a lot better than if someone from infection control comes in and tells them they have to do things a certain way."

Sage thinks PD is easier to sustain than other initiatives.

"A lot of times, solutions are imported from the outside. They are adopted, and then people go back to their usual behaviors. With positive deviance, so many people are involved that if someone slacks off, somebody else will question them. It keeps everybody diligent."

Dr Lloyd emphasizes that positive deviance "is for those problems that simply haven't yielded to the standard approach to improvement," especially if a behavior change is required.

"With health care-acquired infections, our experience has indicated that these are not primarily technical or knowledge problems but behavior problems." ❖

—*Pat Patterson*

References

Association for Professionals in Infection Control and Epidemiology. Guide to the elimination of Methicillin-resistant *Staphylococcus aureus* (MRSA) transmission in hospital settings. Washington, DC: APIC, 2007. www.apic.org

Bradley E H, Curry L A, Ramanadhan S, et al. Research in action: Using positive deviance to improve quality of health care. *Implement Sci.* 2009;4:25.

Healthcare Infection Control Practices Advisory Committee. Management of Multidrug-resistant organisms in healthcare settings, 2006. Atlanta, GA: CDC, 2006. www.cdc.gov/ncidod/dhqp/pdf/ar/mdroGuideline2006.pdf

Lindberg C, Clancy T R. Positive deviance: An elegant solution to a complex problem. *J Nurs Adm.* 2010;40:150-153.

Lloyd J, Buscell P, Lindberg C. Staff-driven cultural transformation diminishes MRSA. *Prevention Strategist.* 2008;1(Spring):10-15.

Pascale R, Sternin J, Sternin M. *The Power of Positive Deviance: How Unlikely Innovators Solve the World's Toughest Problems.* Watertown, MA: Harvard Business Press, 2010.

Ellingson K, Iverson N, Zuckerman J M. SHEA abstract: Multi-center prevention effort significantly cuts MRSA. March 23, 2009. www.plexusinstitute.org/news-events/show_news.cfm?id=1665

Toth M M. Approaching the challenge of eliminating MRSA transmission using positive deviance. PowerPoint. www.apic.org/Content/NavigationMenu/Education/OnlineLearning/Webinars/070124_norstrand.pdf

This article originally appeared in OR Manager, *May 2011;27:1,20-23.*

II. Dashboards and More

OR Dashboards: A Useful Tool for Telling a Story Through Data

Word has traveled to the executive suite that a high percentage of the OR's cases are starting late. There are also rumors of 1½ hour turnover times. As the manager, you know these don't reflect the OR's actual performance. How can you demonstrate that?

One option is a dashboard that tracks key metrics. An OR dashboard can serve as a management tool that tracks the department's performance, tells the OR's story to senior leadership, and spots trends in areas that need improvement. Attributes of an ideal dashboard are described in a new article by Kyung W. Park, MD, MBA, and colleagues from Ohio State University and the University of Vermont (sidebar).

For a dashboard to be successful, the foundation needs to be laid. Metrics need to be selected carefully, data must be reliable, and resources must be allocated to maintain the dashboard.

Starting a conversation

As a management tool, a dashboard is a way "to start a conversation. You want to talk about an issue and drive it to a different place," says Renae Battié, MN, RN, CNOR, regional director of perioperative services for Franciscan Health System, Tacoma, Washington.

She and Steve Alley, MPH, RN, administrative director of surgical service lines at Seattle Children's Hospital, shared tips on dashboards at the fall 2010 Managing Today's OR Suite Conference in Orlando.

Speaking from their 30 years of experience in management, Battié and Alley discussed what they've learned from successful, and not so successful, dashboard efforts.

Here's their advice.

What's your objective?

Decide what purpose you want the dashboard to serve and who the audience will be. Do you need to make the OR's case to senior executives? Do you want to guide the OR's operational performance? Are you on a mission to improve clinical quality?

A dashboard is a way to tell the OR's story. For example, by tracking on-time starts, the dashboard can provide facts for guiding discussions past rumors and anecdotes.

A dashboard can help measure progress on clinical goals, such as Surgical Care Improvement Project (SCIP) measures or infection prevention efforts such as the number of cases between surgical site infections for total hip replacements.

Selecting metrics

Key advice—go slow to go fast. Start with a few metrics, and keep it simple.

"Like any project, take time to think about what needs to be accomplished and who needs to be involved," says Alley.

"In our experience, if you push things through too quickly, soon you're back trying to re-solve the same problem. You may lose valuable time and credibility.

Additional suggestions:

- Decide how many metrics you can reasonably obtain data for and manage.
- Use standardized definitions where possible. Examples are AORN's Perioperative Nursing Data Set (PNDS) and the procedural times glossary from the American Association of Clinical Directors, which has definitions for terms such as anesthesia start and room ready.
- Reach consensus in your own organization on definitions for metrics like start time and turnover time. Consensus on definitions is critical for the data to be accepted later.

How good is the data?

Dashboards are typically created in Excel or similar software, with data gleaned from financial reports, the OR information system, and other sources. Identifying the data sources goes hand-in-hand with selecting metrics. Another critical factor is planning the resources to obtain the data and keep it clean and up to date.

"If it's worth doing, it's worth assigning the resources," Alley says. That may mean assigning an analyst or nurse manager with data skills to dashboard maintenance.

If your databases aren't what you'd like them to be, realize that even a low-tech dashboard can be effective.

"A dashboard doesn't have to be fancy to start a conversation," says Battié.

A nurse manager in one OR reports on-time starts on a white board, with stars for on-time surgeons and a skull-and-cross bones for the tardy.

The board gets the physicians' attention and sparks competition, she notes. "The doctors walk by and say, 'Why didn't I get a star today?'"

The drawback is that this type of dashboard doesn't record and report data over time.

7 dashboard attributes

An ideal OR dashboard would:
- be aligned with the overall goals and objectives of the OR and parent institution
- provide accurate contextual and knowledge-driven data
- display information visually so outliers, trends, and key variations can be grasped quickly and lead to alerts and action plans
- present data that is real time or nearly so
- present a logical hierarchy of information with drill-down capability
- be internet- or intranet-based for timely accessibility
- be part of an organization that accepts objective data as the basis for decision making.

Source: Park K Y, Smaltz D, McFadden D, et al. Operating room dashboard. J Surg Res. 2010; 104:294-300.

Balance your metrics

There's a danger in living entirely by the numbers. Having a balanced set of metrics can avoid that problem. One well-known model is the Balanced Scorecard developed by Robert S. Kaplan and David P. Norton of the Harvard Business School in the 1990s. The scorecard adds strategic and quality metrics to the traditional financial metrics for a more balanced view of performance.

For perioperative services, Battié offers these examples of metrics for a balanced OR dashboard:
- clinical outcomes (eg, skin breakdown, incorrect counts)
- operational outcomes (eg, permit signed, case cancellations)
- financial metrics (eg, direct staff cost/OR minute, supply cost/case)
- institutional initiatives (eg, patient satisfaction, surgeon satisfaction).

Display the data effectively

In deciding on the dashboard's format, consider your audience and what's been successful before. A few principles:
- Make it visual. Color graphics like pie charts and line graphs often tell the story better than tables with numbers.

Battié likes the 3-second rule for designing reports: "If someone can't tell what you're saying in 3 seconds, it won't be effective. Try it out on people who aren't familiar with the data—is the story you're trying to tell clear?"
- Print a clear title, date, and metric definitions on every page of dashboard reports.
- Use white space for readability—don't crowd a printed report.
- Determine whether to set minimums and maximums for data to exclude. For example, will you exclude turnover times over 90 minutes as outliers?
- Decide how often the dashboard will be updated, depending on the audience.

Trigger points

Set scores and targets for dashboard metrics "so you will know what you are reaching for," Battié says.

What will be the triggers telling you that you need to take action? Perhaps it's a downward trend away from your goal or a percentage change of 20% or more.

Some dashboards are color coded with green for "in range," yellow for "need to watch," and red for "take action."

Dealing with data denial

Wherever there's data, there's physician skepticism. Some common reactions: "My patients are sicker." "I had some extreme cases." "The data is too old."

Interestingly, says Alley, there seem to be fewer criticisms when the data carries good news than when the news is bad.

Forming partnerships with physicians, being honest about data deficiencies, and identifying opinion leaders are some ways to respond.

"Involve physician leaders so when they are approached by a surgeon, they can help support the data and process," Alley says.

Identifying an opinion leader who understands the data is helpful.

"The data doesn't have to convince all of the doctors. But a few key leaders who understand the data can help drive it," Battié observes.

Physicians tend not to like data that has been interpreted, she adds. "Willingness to show the raw data shows you are willing to partner with them in doing the right thing with the data."

Be transparent

Alley advocates transparency from the beginning. Talk about variability in the data and why it occurs, he advises. Be clear about the level of detail you are able to get, and not get. And be willing to admit mistakes.

"We've all experienced the comment, 'Your data is wrong,'" he notes. "We know it's not always wrong, but sometimes it's incorrect." Perhaps a surgeon's block utilization excluded some cases because they were misclassified in a different specialty. Being candid about such errors helps to build trust.

"A dashboard can help you present data and build trust in the information," he says. "Then maybe you can get to the root cause of issues you are trying to resolve."

High-tech dashboards

More powerful high-tech dashboards that are easier to create are coming. Seattle Children's is starting to use business intelligence software named Tableau (www.tableausoftware.com).

The OR Benchmarks Collaborative, a collaboration between OR Manager, Inc, and McKesson, offers a web-based dashboard with key performance indicators that enables subscribers to drill into their data and benchmark.

Business intelligence software, by one definition, is designed to mine existing databases to report, analyze, and present data in a way that aids decision making. Typically, the software analyzes data stored in databases, such as the OR information system, meaning a dashboard doesn't have to be created and maintained separately.

Tableau, for example, can produce dashboards and reports quickly from several databases or a database and an Excel spreadsheet.

"Tableau is able to point to a large database and 'farm' information about what is going on," Alley says. "We are finding information we didn't even know we needed to know about."

In one example, he had heard complaints that cases in the hospital's new surgery center were running ahead of schedule, so far ahead that teams were often waiting for the next patient.

He used the software to look at the scheduled versus actual case minutes and was quickly able to get a graphic report showing big gaps between the scheduled and actual times. He realized that because cases were scheduled by increments of 10 and 15 minutes, the scheduling system was overestimating the time needed for the center's shorter cases.

"It's a work enhancement tool that allows quicker development of dashboards," he says. "Once you have it developed, you can sustain it without a lot of energy. It's much easier than trying to maintain an Excel dashboard on a monthly basis." ❖

—*Pat Patterson*

References

AACD Glossary of Times Used for Scheduling and Monitoring of Diagnostic and Therapeutic Procedures. In *Perioperative Standards and Recommended Practices*. Denver, CO: AORN, 2010.

Kaplan R S, Norton D P. Balanced scorecard: Measures that drive performance. *Harvard Bus Rev*. January-February 1992, pp 71-79.

Park K Y, Smaltz D, McFadden D, et al. Operating room dashboard. *J Surg Res*. 2010;104:294-300.

This article originally appeared in OR Manager, *February 2011;27:1,6-8.*

Tracking Data, Changing Behavior

Indiana University Hospital in Indianapolis uses its perioperative dashboard both for monitoring key metrics and for behavior change.

"We figure out what we want to measure on a monthly basis," says Patricia Vassell, MBA, RN, CCRN, CNOR, administrative director of surgical services. The department has 24 ORs. Examples of metrics are:

- FTE utilization
- first-case on-time starts
- case cancellations
- PACU admission delays (number of patients who cannot leave the OR when surgery is complete because no PACU bed is available)
- turnover time (patient out to patient in)
- PACU length of stay
- OR utilization (7 am to 3:30 pm)
- total number of cases
- total number of OR hours.

The color-coded dashboard is shared monthly with the OR's leaders, physicians, and nursing staff.

"We post it on the bulletin board every month. Everyone knows what the dashboard is," Vassell says.

Recently, the dashboard helped in addressing late starts for first cases.

"We constantly look to see what is going on," she says. The top 3 reasons for delays get the attention. Initially, it took some effort to make sure nurses documented the delay codes accurately and consistently.

In tackling the top 3 reasons for delays, they identified some nursing issues involving instrumentation and equipment.

Once those were resolved and no longer appeared in the top 3, physician issues rose to the top.

The OR's medical director, Eric Wiebke, MD, MBA, FACS, worked with the OR committee to set expectations for the physicians.

Ultimately, one surgeon lost his first-case time for a month, which turned the issue around. The next month, Vassell says, he began arriving as early as 6 am—much to the staff's surprise.

"Our physician leader has really held the physicians accountable for their performance, and

Top 3 delay reasons

	Aug 2010	Sept 2010	Oct 2010
1.	Surgeon - H&P not completed	Surgeon - H&P not completed	Surgeon - Procedure consent not completed
2.	Tie: All other reasons tied	Patient/family - Questions/ apprehension	Tie: Anesthesia - assessment not completed; surgeon - late/ unavailable
3.	Tie: All other reasons tied	Tie: Anesthesia - assessment not completed; surgeon - late/ unavailable; surgeon - procedure consent not completed	Tie: Preop assessment not completed; surgeon - H&P not completed

Note: Data source is Cognos.
*Excludes add-on rooms, MRI/CT cases, "bumped" cases, living related donors, jump rooms, and schedule/case order change.
Source: Indiana University Hospital.

OR performance

Surgery Dashboard

■ Achieved target
■ Target not achieved; however, improvement from previous month
■ Target not achieved; decreased improvement from previous month

Metric	Metric definition	Measure	Data source/ contact	Target	Aug 10	Sept 10	Oct 10	Status towards target	Trend
FTE utilization	OR staffing levels exceed the flexed workload levels	Comparison between actual and flexed budget	Monthly FTE report	1.0% or less	2.0% under flexed budget	4.89% under flex budget	1.72% over flex budget	Using more FTEs than flex budget allows but decreased variance % from previous month	
First-case starts	Patient in room at scheduled time for first case	% of cases that patient enters the suite no more than 5 minutes after the scheduled start	Cognos	75.0%	95.0%	90.0%	74.0%	Decrease in % of first cases started on time	
Case cancellation rate (excludes transplant)	Number of canceled cases per weekday (excluding transplant)	Number of canceled cases per weekday/total number of cases per weekday (excluding transplant)	Cerner	2.0%	0.82%	1.17%	0.50%	Decreased from previous month	
PACU admission delays	Total number of occurrences and minutes that patient is held in OR	Total number of occurrences and minutes that patient is held in OR for Phase 1	Cerner	0	1 case 32 minutes total	1 case 12 minutes total	3 cases 52 minutes total	Increase in number of minutes patients held in OR	
Turnover time*	Amount of time from when one patient exits an OR until the next patient enters the same OR within 60 minutes	% of cases that are turned over in 30 minutes or less	Cognos	90.0%	73.2%	80.0%	76.0%	Decrease in % of cases turned over in 30 minutes or less	
Length of stay in PACU	Amount of time from admission to discharge in PACU for Phase 1	Time patient enters PACU until discharged from PACU for Phase 1	Cerner	90 min or less	86 minutes	8 minutes	8 minutes	Met target and no change from previous month	
Overall OR utilization	# of actual OR hours used/# of OR hours available 7:30a-3:30p	# of actual OR hours used/# of OR hours available 7:30a-3:30p	Cerner	85.0%	65.5%	62.2%	62.8%	Increase in hours OR is used between 7:30a-3:30p	
# of cases			Cognos		1,004	995	1,064		
# of surg hours			Cognos		3,180	3,016	2,936		

*Turnover time excludes pm cases, jump rooms, add-on rooms, bumped cases, and "previous case ended early." Source: Indiana University.

that has made a difference," Vassell says. "We have had days where 100% of our cases were on time."

She adds: "Everything is driven by the dashboard. I find physicians will respond if you can show them the data.

"Without data, it's just finger pointing."

Dashboard summary

Audience: Medical and nursing staffs and perioperative leaders

Metrics: FTE utilization, on-time first-case starts, and other operational metrics

Frequency: Monthly

Software: Dashboard is in Excel. Data source is nurses' documentation in the perioperative information system. ❖

This article originally appeared in OR Manager, *February 2011;27:10-11.*

III. Governance

Is Your OR Leadership Team Up to Health Care Reform Challenges?

How can you make progress on on-time starts? Are you attracting the right cases to meet your volume and revenue projections? How can you manage block utilization more consistently?

The first answer to these persistent questions is good OR governance and a strong leadership team built on collaboration among nursing, surgery, and anesthesia.

That firm foundation will be critical as the nation moves into health care reform. With tightening Medicare and Medicaid reimbursement and higher stakes for quality reporting and performance, ORs will need to be in top form. Though insurance coverage will expand and bring more paying patients to hospitals, many of those patients will be covered by government programs with low reimbursement. Medicare and Medicaid will also move toward value-based purchasing, or pay for performance, starting in 2013, tying a small part of hospitals' DRG payments to quality and efficiency measures.

Is the traditional OR Committee up to the task? If the committee meets sporadically, has trouble raising a quorum, and is mainly a forum for complaints, it's time to look at another model.

Two consultants described governance models that can place the OR on a firm foundation to meet the challenges ahead. In the next article, 2 hospitals describe their governance structures and what they believe makes them effective.

OR as asset

Perioperative services are a major asset—a multimillion-dollar business—that needs to be guided by a board of directors, advises Mary Jane Edwards, RN, MHSA, CNOR, FACHE, of Deloitte Consulting, McLean, Virginia.

"The OR contributes 65% of the margin for a hospital—it's your revenue engine," she says, adding that a business of that magnitude needs a structure like that of any successful business.

The 12- to 15-member board is an operation that takes an interest in the whole perioperative enterprise.

"It's like being on the board of a public company," says Edwards, a former OR director who has been consulting with surgical services departments for 15 years. "A director can't just be interested in his or her own division. Directors need to act together to protect the shared asset, perioperative services."

Day-to-day management of the department is carried out by a management team that reports to the governing board. The team, which includes a nurse administrator, anesthesiologist, and surgeon, reports to the board and interprets and executes the board's policies.

Who are the members?

The board consists of respected representatives from surgery, anesthesia, nursing, and the administration, with members selected based on criteria, not title.

"What's important is that the surgeons and anesthesiologists on the board really have an understanding and investment in the OR running well," Edwards says.

The hospital administrator directly responsible for perioperative services should be an active participant.

"This can't be just an honorific appointment," she adds. "The administration brings the larger picture and provides support."

What happens to the traditional OR committee?

Some hospitals redirect the OR committee's charge in line with the model described for perioperative governance, says Edwards. Others redirect the committee's charge, perhaps to focus on issues like morbidity and mortality, specific safety issues, and outreach to community physicians and surgeons.

Clear expectations

Expectations for the board of directors need to be clear. The mission should be set forth in the board's charter, Edwards advises. The board should be familiar with the hospital's strategic mission, determine the OR's key performance indicators, ensure resources are available to fulfill the mission, and track performance.

The aim is to set specific targets for improvement, which many hospitals are doing through methods like Lean Six Sigma.

"With perioperative governance, there is no place to hide. You have to achieve the goals," she says. She suggests a set of clear, basic indicators. Examples are:
- OR utilization
- first case on-time starts
- turnover time
- case volume and case hours
- quality and safety measures

- recruitment goals
- length of stay in the postanesthesia care unit.

Active members

The board needs active, participating members. "Make this the one committee that members attend if they can't attend any other," she suggests. That may mean re-evaluating the committee assignments of key physicians.

Regular attendance is expected. Some boards set a rule: Members who are absent 3 times per year or for 3 consecutive meetings are automatically replaced by another member who will be actively engaged.

Regarding compensation, Edwards says that in her experience, physicians have not requested supplemental payment for serving on the perioperative governing body.

"The reason is that this committee is so important," she says. It decides on the rules for block scheduling, the hours of operation, and other policies that directly affect physicians' practices.

"Rather than a stipend, their payoff is in the creation of a disciplined, effective, and safe environment for their patients, families, and practice."

Surgery executive committee

A similar model that works well for any size of department, whether a 50-OR academic medical center or a 2-OR rural hospital, has 3 components, says Randy Heiser, president and CEO of Sullivan Healthcare Consulting, Ann Arbor, Michigan, which specializes in perioperative consulting:

- A surgery executive committee, typically a duo or triad with a nurse administrator and an anesthesiologist and/or a surgeon. "They run the OR and enforce policy," he says.
- A surgical services committee that acts as a board of directors, with the executive committee members as cochairs. This is an operational committee, not a medical staff committee, and reports to the CEO.
- A broad-based medical staff communication plan to convey information directly from the committee to the medical staff. The plan might include a regular town hall meeting or news bulletin.

In most hospitals where Heiser has consulted, the physician members of the surgery executive committee are paid positions. In a small hospital, the positions might be a part of an FTE, whereas in a large facility, they are generally full-time.

Good of the program

The physician members of the executive committee aren't necessarily the chief of surgery and chief of anesthesia, Heiser points out. The key is whether they are willing to step outside their specialty and make decisions based on the good of the program.

That's in contrast to the traditional OR committee where the members typically have been selected by the medical staff and "felt they owned the OR, and

OR governance success factors

Support from senior management

Support from the top of the organization is "absolutely the one thing that makes governing bodies more or less effective," says Randy Heiser of Sullivan Healthcare Consulting.

"If the CEO who talks with an angry surgeon says anything other than, 'I will make sure to get you in front of the right committee so you can get this resolved,' it's dead in the water."

Clear responsibilities

Responsibilities and accountability for the OR board of directors and executive committee need to be clearly outlined.

"Once you tell a surgeon you don't know whom to take an issue to, the surgeon will solve it independently, and you will no longer have a governance structure," he says.

The right members

- Are the members able to think about what is best for the program rather than only about what is best for themselves or their own service?
- Is there a balance among surgery, nursing, and anesthesia so all 3 groups participate and have a say?

the OR was there as a service to the surgeons. That can create problems with anesthesia, because the traditional OR committee doesn't have anesthesia providers present," he notes.

Clear expectations are established. In a department that is working well, the executive committee might focus on strategic planning and operational and financial performance. In an OR that is implementing new programs, efforts might be directed toward those issues, compliance with policies, and so forth.

"Overall, this committee has to be fully responsible for the daily operations of the perioperative program. How that is defined is up to each hospital," he says.

Direct communication

As part of the plan, Heiser recommends a direct communication route with the OR medical staff. "Leaving it up to the chiefs to communicate with their services doesn't work."

One option is physician forums or town hall meetings, typically held quarterly unless there are pressing issues.

"It's a way for the executives to speak directly to the medical staff and give them an opportunity to have input that isn't filtered through anyone else," he says.

A typical agenda for a town hall meeting might include:
- the latest OR metrics
- issues and changes facing the department
- a "first reading" and feedback on new policies being considered
- new business and concerns.

These governance structures are easier to implement than they were 3 years ago, Heiser observes.

"Surgeons are starting to see in other hospitals that this does work," he says. "They see that with a good governance structure and good physician leadership, the volume of cases goes up, the money available to invest in new equipment and technology goes up, and most surgeons are doing more procedures." Sometimes, physicians who have been the greatest skeptics become the biggest converts.

"They see they are better off with the new model," Heiser says. ❖

—*Pat Patterson*

This article originally appeared in OR Manager, *June 2010;26:1,6-7.*

OR Governance Builds A Strong Foundation

Two hospitals, both recognized nationally for their strong performance on patient outcome and financial measures, describe their approaches to OR governance.

Leadership triad provides a strong base for safety

Regions Hospital
St Paul, Minnesota
Level 1 trauma center with 17 ORs and an ambulatory surgery center

As Regions Hospital moved to a greater emphasis on patient safety, its OR leaders realized they needed a stronger foundation.

"When we started talking about patient safety, we realized we had some work to do," says the senior director of surgical services, Dana Langness, RN, BSN, MA.

Their response was to form a leadership triad with a surgeon, anesthesiologist, and the senior director of surgical services.

Regions is part of Minnesota-based HealthPartners, a nonprofit integrated health system known for its cost-effectiveness and quality. HealthPartners's CEO, Mary Brainerd, has been a leader in the Institute for Healthcare Improvement's Triple Aim, which seeks to improve the patient's experience with care, the health of the population, and the cost of care.

In 2009, Regions was rated as one of the nation's 45 "high value" hospitals by the Leapfrog Group for its performance on complex high-risk procedures.

OR governing body

The leadership triad includes David Dries, MD, a surgeon and assistant medical director for surgical care; Matt Layman, MD, an anesthesiologist and medical director of perioperative services; and Langness.

"It was our request that it be structured this way," says Langness. "We are mentoring a partnership, which is a huge change. People have not been taught in school how to collaborate at the level necessary to keep our patients safe."

The triad reports to the senior hospital leadership; Drs Dries and Layman also report to the vice president for medical affairs. About 80% of the physicians are employed by HealthPartners.

The three meet quarterly with Brainerd to give a quality update, including the status of the Surgical Care Improvement Project (SCIP), infection rates, retained foreign bodies, and other issues.

"As a result, the team feels supported in their work and personally accountable," Langness says.

OR committee's role

An OR committee, part of the medical staff structure, meets quarterly and includes the surgeon service line leaders as well as Langness and other participants. The committee reviews surgical volume, block utilization, a quality update, any new policies needing approval, concerns about policy compliance, and other issues. A subgroup consisting of Langness, the service line director, the OR business manager, and if necessary a surgeon leader meets regularly to review block utilization and report to the OR committee.

A separate safety task force meets biweekly. Results are shared at regular joint physician-staff in-services.

Leave titles at door

"We actually get people together in a room so we can learn at the same time," Langness says.

"We always start the in-services with a story—with a good catch, an award we have received, or something to elicit passion and the idea that we are all here together for patient safety. We leave our titles at the door. The surgical tech's opinion is just as important as the surgeon's opinion."

The patient safety focus extends to physician and staff recruitment.

"When we hire new physicians and staff, we are looking for people who are passionate about making a difference for their patients and health care," Langness says. "We want people who are going to push us to the next level."

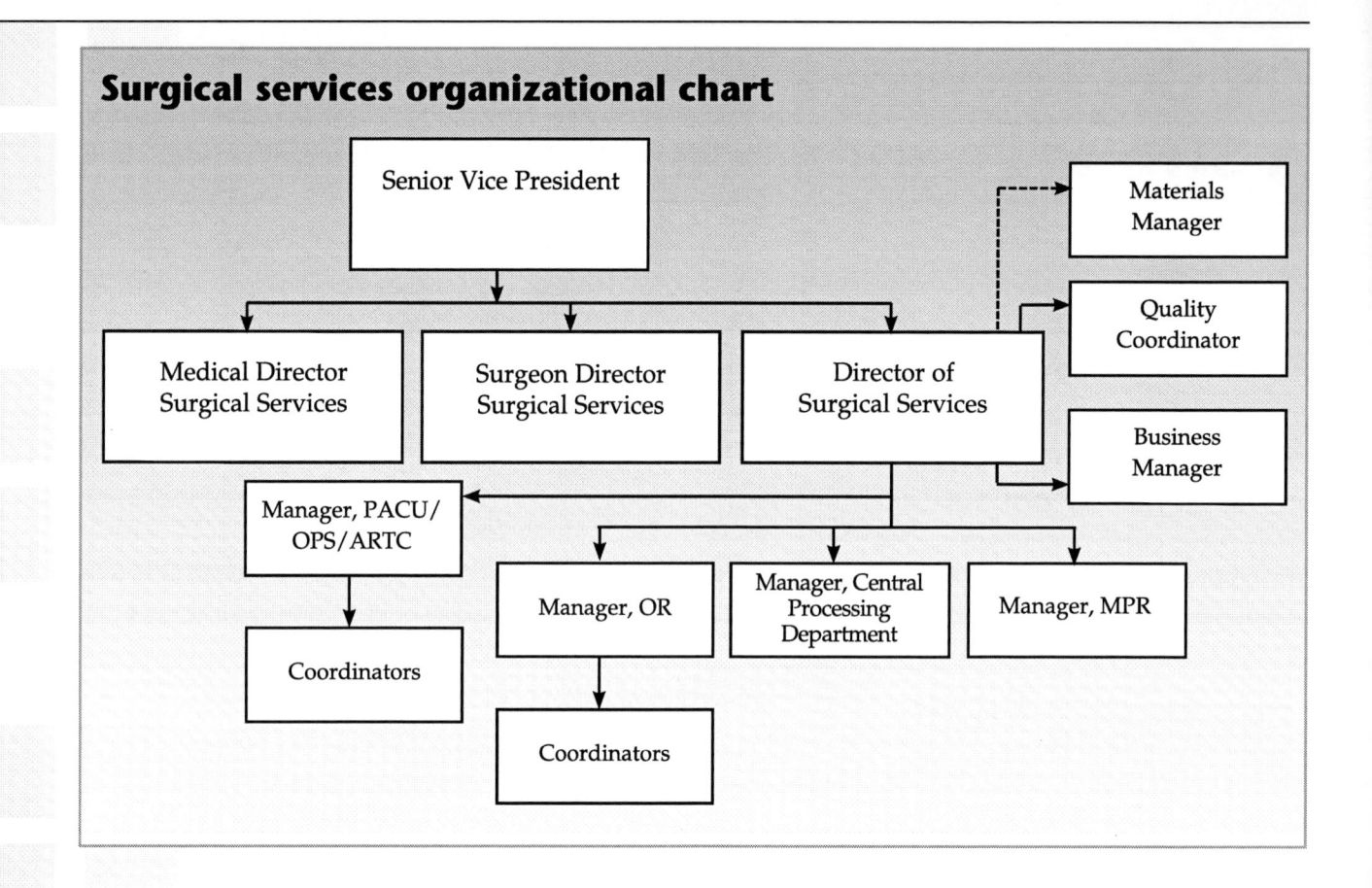

Surgical services organizational chart

```
                    Senior Vice President
                           │
        ┌──────────────────┼──────────────────┐────────── Materials Manager
        │                  │                  │                │
  Medical Director    Surgeon Director   Director of ──────── Quality Coordinator
  Surgical Services   Surgical Services  Surgical Services
                                              │─────────── Business Manager
        ┌─────────────────────┬───────────────┼───────────────┐
   Manager, PACU/         Manager, OR    Manager, Central  Manager, MPR
   OPS/ARTC                               Processing
        │                      │          Department
   Coordinators            Coordinators
```

A surgeon joins OR exec committee

Munson Medical Center
Traverse City, Michigan
Nonprofit regional referral center with 14 ORs

Munson is one of 23 hospitals in the country to earn the Everest Award from the Thomson Reuters's 100 Top Hospitals program for its performance and long-term improvements. Munson also won the American Hospital Association-McKesson Quest for Quality Prize in 2009. It is a Magnet hospital for nursing excellence and participates in the American College of Surgeons National Surgical Quality Improvement Program (NSQIP). Most of the physicians are in private practice.

OR governing body

The governing body, called the OR executive committee, recently added a third member, a general and vascular surgeon. The 3 members now include the medical director of surgical services, anesthesiologist Robert Cline, MD; the director of surgical services, Maxine Hunter, RN, MSN; and Walter Noble, MD, as the surgeon director of surgical services.

The committee reports to a senior vice president (chart). Drs Cline and Noble also have reporting relationships to the vice president for medical affairs. Dr Cline's position is 50% administrative and 50% clinical. Dr Noble's is 20% administrative and 80% clinical. Neither is the chief of service.

An 8- to 10-member surgery committee serves in an advisory capacity and is part of the medical staff structure. Members include surgeon representatives, Hunter; the OR manager, Loie Rainey, RN; and the senior vice president.

Responsibilities

Hunter has administrative responsibility for the OR and related departments. Dr Cline manages the block schedule, monitors performance indicators, communicates with the surgery committee and medical staff, and handles day-to-day interactions with physicians. Dr Noble heads Munson's NSQIP project. He also provides representation for the surgeons on the OR executive committee.

The executive committee enforces policies such as those for block scheduling, management of the block schedule, and urgent and emergent cases.

Of his role, Dr Noble says, "It has been helpful for the surgical specialties to feel they have input. It's another set of eyes."

Hunter adds that having a surgeon member of the leadership team has been especially helpful in situations such as the late afternoon when cases are running late, and decisions are needed about which cases will go next. Dr Cline adds that Dr Noble provides important input regarding the purchase of capital equipment and new technology.

"It's been a huge support to have the two specialties represented, especially when you have conflict situations," Hunter says. "It is great to have a surgeon available to represent the surgeons, to have anesthesia involved, and to have all 3 perspectives." ❖

This article originally appeared in OR Manager, *June 2010;26:8-10.*

A Lean Process For OR Technology

With tighter budgets and long lists of technology requests, organizations need a fair and systematic way to set priorities. At Virginia Mason Medical Center (VMMC) in Seattle, where Lean manufacturing principles are part of the culture, it was natural to apply Lean to the review of new surgical supplies and technology.

The existing process was more like "a speed bump to yes," Steve Schaefer, vice president for finance, told OR Manager.

The new more robust process, which includes a more active role for physicians, also takes less time, 15 to 16 days compared to 45 days before.

Previously, new product requests were submitted using an online form to the purchasing department. The purchasing department gathered the information it could and forwarded the request to the appropriate VP, who often held the request, awaiting more information. The requesting physician would pressure the VP, who would generally say yes. The 45 days left physicians tapping their feet, and there was little coordination with other departments, such as finance.

The new process helps to build consensus among specialists and to align technology acquisitions with the organization's goals (sidebar). Schaefer estimated the improvements will yield supply cost savings of $1 million in 2009, about 1% to 2% of its supply spend. Costs will also be avoided because of items not purchased.

Leader in Lean

VMMC, a nonprofit integrated delivery network, is a national leader for Lean in health care, having embraced the Toyota-pioneered approach to quality improvement in 2000.

"It's the water we swim in," Schaefer, says. Simply stated, in a Lean culture, everyone strives to eliminate waste and inefficiency. All VMMC personnel are trained in Lean, including the physician CEO Gary S. Kaplan, MD, other senior executives, and physicians. Many travel to Japan for 2 weeks to observe Lean in action.

Bringing physicians in

All of the stakeholders realized product review needed improvement. Because most technology requests come from physicians, VMMC needed a way to bring them into the process.

Two major steps were to:
- create a supply chain oversight team
- hire a physician advisor.

The oversight team, described in a report from the Health Care Financial Management Association, Engaging Physicians for Supply Chain Savings, includes not only senior executives but also the chief medical officer, medical director, and physician advisor.

The team's role is to maximize the value of the supply chain by ensuring all materials are used effectively and processes are cost-efficient. Having physicians on the oversight team creates a sense of ownership in the supply chain, Schaefer said. Rather than being viewed as a separate department dictating policy, the supply chain "gets enterprise commitment and accountability," he said.

A physician advisor

The second major step was to enlist a senior orthopedic surgeon, Paul Benca, MD, as the physician advisor to serve as a bridge between the administrators and physicians.

"I can go back and forth between the camps so we have good communication," he says. His position is split between clinical and administrative duties.

Dr Benca says he can go to the physicians and ask for more information about their requests. He also brings the physicians information about costs and discusses how the purchase fits with the organization's objectives.

"A lot of the section heads—including myself as head of the orthopedics section—weren't even aware of products our staff members were requesting," Dr Benca said.

"I think physicians understand the need to be good stewards. If you give them examples of what things are going to cost, they can make a better choice."

Breaking down walls

Dr Benca has worked to break down walls between specialties to help get consensus on technology decisions. This is one improvement that came out of a rapid process improvement workshop on the product review process. The workshops are short, intense projects that bring a team together to improve a process.

Three surgeons were involved in the product review workshop, along with nurses and administrative staff from radiology, cardiology, and gastroenterology,

"You need a breadth of people in the room," says Schaefer. "It's eye-opening when you realize how each section deals with its own issues."

To make it easier for physicians to participate, VMMC sometimes shortens the workshops to 1 or 2 days rather than the usual 5 days. That's possible, Dr Benca notes, because physicians already have a background in Lean.

He also brought together physicians from technology-intensive areas—gastroenterology, interventional radiology, and the OR—to find out what they expect from the process. They, in turn, asked their sections. He learned that physicians wanted a process that is:

- reasonably quick
- nimble
- uses an electronic request form.

Single-site laparoscopic surgery

Laparoscopic equipment is a popular but pricey request, particularly for general surgery, urology, and gynecology. Two recent requests had annual price tags of $100,000 with no increase in reimbursement.

To help vet these requests, Dr Benca formed an ad hoc task force of representatives from each specialty. VMMC is conducting a trial on single-incision laparoscopic surgery, new instrumentation that allows surgeons to operate through a single incision in the umbilicus.

"The questions are, 'Is it worth what it is going to cost us? Does it really add anything?'" Dr Benca says. "We will go back after the trial to see if it makes sense to the requesters and ask them to justify the expense."

A plan for implants

Dr Benca plans to meet soon with the orthopedics section to review implant selection for hip and knee replacements. Part of the new approach will be to share implant costs with the physicians, which VMMC previously did not do.

Implant pricing does not seem to be an issue. "We have found through outside parties that our costs for orthopedic prostheses and cardiac implants are very competitive," he says.

Dr Benca plans to lead a cost analysis of newer approaches to treating joints, including partial knee replacements, hip resurfacing, and newer types of implants such as ceramic-on-ceramic components.

"We are going to look at the true costs of these products with the discounts and what our payers pay," he says. "I think that will help our physicians make intelligent choices to do what is best for patients but also try to keep the costs under control."

Strengthening product review

Improvements that helped Virginia Mason's product review to become leaner and more robust:

Added expertise

More expertise was added to the product review team, including clinical experts and representatives from the finance department, chargemaster and coding units as well as purchasing and contracting. Dr Benca brings the physicians' voice. VMMC's group purchasing organization, Amerinet, lends data analysis and benchmarking expertise.

Clearing requests

- A short section was added to the product request form requiring physicians who submit a request to justify the purchase and to clear the request with their section heads.
- Section heads review the request and discuss it with section members to see how the technology fits with the specialty's needs. They are encouraged to ask: "Can everybody in the section use this product? Does it allow us to do something we couldn't do before? Is it strategically important for the program?"

Financial analysis

The product review team must gather complete information about the product before forwarding the request to the finance office for review.

Product trials

The team encourages product trials. "We are happy to approve trials," Dr Benca says. "Trials can be very helpful."

Schaefer and Dr Benca stress the product review process is a work in progress.

"The whole concept behind Lean methodology is one of continuous change and improvement," Schaefer says. "The process to eliminate waste never ends."

Breaking down the walls among specialties for technology decisions has been a major improvement "that will pay dividends year after year," Schaefer says. ❖

—*Pat Patterson*

This article originally appeared in OR Manager, *April 2010;26:20-21.*

V. Physician Preference Items

Top Strategies for Juggling Quantity, Cost of Physician Preference Items

Managing the costs of procedures with implants continues to be a juggling act for OR directors and business managers.

Total joint replacements, once profitable, have seen prices climb while Medicare reimbursement slides. Some spinal procedures still have a positive margin because the surgery is more often performed in younger patients with commercial insurance. But financial success depends on an organization's ability to work with the surgeons to control costs.

ROi (Resource Optimization and Innovation) is the supply chain arm for the 20-hospital Sisters of Mercy Health System based in St Louis. ROi's mission is to improve the clinical, operational, and financial performance of customers through a clinically integrated supply chain.

"The Sisters of Mercy is all about reduction of variation and improved efficiencies because we believe that drives safety and quality," says Marita Parks, RN, MHA, ROi's vice president for performance consulting.

Here are ROi's top strategies for physician preference items.

Develop a compelling reason for change

For a hospital or health system to enlist physicians' support for managing sensitive items like orthopedic and spinal implants, there must be a compelling reason for change that goes beyond finances, Parks advises.

"Three critical factors have to be there—clinical, operational, as well as financial. We ask, 'What are the opportunities that go along with better management of the process?'"

For example, if the number of implant vendors is reduced, will that help to improve operational processes? Fewer vendors could help reduce variation, which should lead to a more streamlined, safer process.

"If you say the reason you want to reduce variation is to improve patient safety and help provide better service to the surgeons—and by the way, we are going to reduce some costs—that is more compelling than just saying, 'We have to save money,'" she says.

Have senior leaders commit to the process

Sisters of Mercy has a hospital CEO council that meets monthly. Projects with a large impact, such as addressing physician preference items, are presented to the council so the CEOs can discuss opportunities and strategies for involving physicians and other key stakeholders.

"We keep them in the loop as we work through the process," Parks says. As the project progresses, she and her team work with the CEOs to develop talking points to assist them in discussions with physicians who have questions or concerns.

Develop a strategy to reduce variation

ROi uses 2 approaches for reducing variation in use of physician preference items:
- capitation
- vendor compression.

Both require a great deal of collaboration with physicians.

The most effective strategy, Parks says, has been to reduce the number of vendors, termed "vendor compression." This strategy accomplishes the twin objectives of reducing variation and reducing cost by driving volume to fewer vendors.

There has been debate about which method is the most effective. Reducing the number of implant vendors is difficult because surgeons are reluctant to give up a product line they are accustomed to and have a strong loyalty to. On the other hand, with capitation, surgeons continue to use any vendor they choose, and the hospital and vendors agree to ceiling prices for implant classes or constructs. Capitation has less impact on clinical practice and operations than vendor compression.

"Capitation can work," Parks says. "You need significant buy-in from physicians because if you have vendors who will not participate in the capitated pricing and physicians continue to use those vendors, costs increase and the capitation model does not work. Physicians must agree to align with us by telling vendors that only if they participate will the surgeons use their products."

In ROi's experience, after benchmarking among its 20 hospitals and comparing best practices, limiting the number of vendors has been more successful than capitation.

"It is not always the most popular strategy, but it works. It both saves costs and reduces variability," she says.

With fewer vendors, the staff has fewer types of instrument sets to manage. This is no small matter because a major orthopedic case can take 15 or more trays. With fewer types of trays, the staff can become

With technology, strategy shifting to 'If you prove it, they will come'

What's going to bring patients to your facility for spine care? One factor has been whether you offer the latest technology—minimally invasive surgery, computer-guided navigation, the latest CT scanner.

The theme has been, "If you buy it, they will come." The new theme is, "If you prove it, they will come."

Demonstrating performance is becoming a way to differentiate your organization from competitors.

"Success will be less about what technology you have and more about how well you use it," says Steve Miff, PhD, vice president with Sg2, Skokie, Illinois, a consulting firm focused on health care strategy and business development.

Can you demonstrate how your organization is doing on measures like reoperation and readmission rates? Will you be able to show your services yield better outcomes and a faster return to normal activities?

Health care facilities will become more selective in the technology they pick, Miff says. "They will focus more on the impact of that technology—not only on market differentiation but also on how it affects clinical performance, operations, and costs of care."

That will require more consensus on measurements, more robust data systems, and the ability to collect data across different sites.

Here are some trends Miff sees for orthopedics and spine care.

More transparency

At least 1 million patients covered by WellPoint, one of the nation's largest insurers, can now look up ratings on their physician from Zagat, best known for rating restaurants. They can see how other patients rate their physician on trust, communication, availability, and environment.

Clinical data is also available, though it's still limited. Patients can check Medicare's Hospital Compare website to see how hospitals in their area are doing on measures like administering antibiotics before surgery and venous thromboembolism prophylaxis. WebMD, Health Grades, the Leapfrog group, and others also offer reports.

Patients shopping for services

Consumers are starting to use this information to make decisions about their care, and they will demand more data, Miff says.

On spine care, for example, patients still want access to the most innovative care. But they also want solid information on treatment options, both surgical and medical care.

"I think we'll see more patients shopping for services, and I think we will see this play out first in orthopedics and spine," Miff says. "It's early, but it is a trend that is going to accelerate."

Progressive organizations are already collecting data and posting it on their web sites so they can communicate directly with patients and physicians.

Bundled hospital, MD payment

Medicare is experimenting with a new program called ACE—the Acute Care Episode demonstration project—which gives a single global payment to a hospital and physicians for certain orthopedic and cardiac procedures. The government hopes this will encourage hospitals and physicians to collaborate in improving quality and managing costs. The demo will take place in Texas, Oklahoma, New Mexico, and Colorado.

"This is the way payment is evolving, looking at a bundled payment for a broader continuum of care," Miff says.

Need for better data systems

These efforts will require more and better data. Systems are needed to capture and connect spine care data on spine care across settings, including the hospital, surgery center, surgeons' offices, diagnostic center, and physical therapy clinic.

These systems are in their infancy, and comparison data are lacking. In cardiovascular services, Miff says, 85% of Sg2's client hospitals use national benchmarking data. But in orthopedics, only about 30% are using national data, and another 30% are using regional data. The other 40% just use their "best estimates."

Also needed is consensus on measurements. What kind of data should organizations be collecting?

"Spine programs should be collecting procedure-specific data," Miff advises. That includes clinical outcomes, operational performance, financials, and staff and physician performance. Data are also needed matching patients' severity of illness to outcomes. Other measures should include where applicable length of stay, cost of implants as a percentage of reimbursement, discharge disposition, return-to-work time, complications, readmissions, and improvements in functional scores.

"Then they will be able to review the data and develop processes to address measures they want to improve," he says. "They will also be able to look back and match certain procedures and implants to patient types and be able to assess what produced superior results."

Programs that are successful are starting slow and taking small steps. For example, they might start by collecting data for patients having laminectomy or discectomy by a subgroup of surgeons.

But a wider view is needed. Miff says Sg2 is developing metrics for data collection that would enable benchmarking and practice comparisons. Sg2 is working with other organizations, including the National Spine Network (NSN) and Priority Consult, a company that develops software systems for patient management.

NSN, a nonprofit spine registry based in Marietta, Georgia, has gathered spine data for use by physician practices and research centers. To automate data collection, NSN has software called SpineChart that allows patients and physicians to use touch screens to record information about care. Though the software is currently focused on physician practices, NSN plans to expand it to hospitals. For more information, visit www.nationalspinenetwork.org or phone 404/520-1555.

How will trends affect ORs?

What impact will these trends have on technology decisions for surgery?

"I think teams will be more aware of the implications of adding something new," Miff comments. With performance transparency, more profiling will be done, not only for individual surgeons but also for whole programs and departments.

"If you have a surgeon who is extremely aggressive with new technology and new procedures, but the surgeon's readmission rates are high, that will affect the whole department because the whole department will be profiled."

He thinks performance data will become part of the conversation with surgeons about new technology.

"It will make it easier to counsel caution and take a more comprehensive look at the impact of a new procedure or technology before it is adopted," he says. "There will be a need to understand the impact on staffing and the operation of the facility as well as the broad clinical impact."

Physicians are data driven, and as data becomes more refined, working with physicians to develop programs and make technology decisions will become more targeted and productive, he predicts.

---

more proficient at reprocessing and setting up cases, improving service to surgeons.

This strategy is consistent with the Sisters of Mercy's overall approach of improving quality by using protocols or standardized methods for everything that makes sense in improving patient care.

"That way, care providers have a consistent roadmap for producing predictable outcomes," Parks says.

In the Sisters of Mercy total joint initiative, the number of orthopedic vendors was reduced from 13 to 5, shifting market share and achieving better pricing from the remaining vendors, she says. The 5 final vendors were market leaders across the system, and the vast majority of surgeons either used one of them or had in the past.

Enlist physician leaders

The secret to vendor compression is enlisting a respected physician leader. Says Parks, "If a physician leads these initiatives, the rate of success is much higher."

ROi is currently conducting an initiative on bone products used in spinal surgery, where physician leadership is instrumental.

"First, we try to understand the utilization of these products and what the opportunities are," she explains. "Then we try to find an influential surgeon who can talk with peers" to help reach consensus on the products and vendors that will be used based on criteria the surgeons have identified, such as quality, safety, and costs.

"What we have found in particular with surgeons is that peer-to-peer communication and support are the most successful strategies," she says.

Ideally, the physician leader will be a practicing surgeon in the same specialty. "Physicians tend to listen to peers who understand their day-to-day challenges," she says. To be effective, physician leaders also need strong leadership and financial skills.

Align incentives

With physicians under growing financial pressure in their own practices, they may have little time or inclination to help on these projects. Parks says there are incentives hospitals can offer that are within the law and not overly expensive.

"People tend to say, 'There's little we can do,'" she says. "But I think there are things you can offer surgeons that are appealing and don't cost a lot of money. We try to find out what the drivers are with specific physician groups. The key is active engagement of the physicians in the process."

Orthopedic surgeons, for example, may want another C-arm for the operating room.

"We would need to first validate the need for this equipment. Then we could collaborate with the physicians to develop a target for reducing implant variation and cost," she explains. The savings could then be earmarked for purchase of the preapproved equipment.

A longer term goal might be to work with the surgeons on improving their quality of work life through OR efficiencies such as on-time starts and shorter turnover times. Another incentive might be an offer to pay a physician leader for administrative time to lead the project. Such arrangements must, of course, be based on fair-market value and avoid violating the federal Anti-kickback Statute, which prohibits remuneration in exchange for referrals or for recommending purchase of supplies and services that are reimbursable under government health programs.

Draw on physician-to-physician comparisons

Presenting surgeons with data on their individual practice patterns for a particular procedure can be an effective way to focus their attention on implant and supply utilization.

"There are lots of opportunities if you're willing to dig into the data," Parks says.

"When we do these physician-to-physician comparisons, they are always blinded. We show them the variability between Drs A, B, C, and D. We say, 'These are some of the drivers of variability in your practice.' That's often an eye opener to them. They will say, 'Oh, I use this device, and nobody else uses it?'"

Develop a vendor credentialing program

Sisters of Mercy is implementing an enterprisewide vendor access and credentialing system for its 20 hospitals. The systems will require vendors to be registered and meet certain criteria, depending on their level of patient contact.

Parks sees this as a necessary part of providing a safe environment, meeting regulatory requirements, protecting patients' privacy, and reducing the infection risk.

Senior executives are being educated about the process so they can explain the program to physicians and vendors. Then if a vendor complains to a CEO about "being locked out of the OR," the CEO can explain, "It's not that we're locking you out. But there are criteria that must be followed and qualifications that must be met.

"Again, this is engaging the key stakeholders in the initiatives and partnering with them to accomplish established goals," Parks comments. ❖

This article originally appeared in OR Manager, *January 2009;25:1,8-9,13.*

VI. Preoperative Process

How Clinics Help The Preop Process

The preoperative process is critical to safe care and a smooth OR process. Missing paperwork, incomplete assessments, and the need for last-minute consults can disrupt any surgical day.

Is a preoperative clinic the answer? Each organization needs to weigh the cost against the potential benefits, such as fewer delays and cancellations and improved reimbursement through more accurate coding of patients' comorbidities. Clinics also help to ensure regulatory requirements and payer guidelines are met.

OR Manager spoke with leaders of 3 preoperative clinics, each with a different format, who say the clinics have made the presurgical assessment process more efficient and consistent.

Standardizing the assessment

The preop clinic at Brigham & Women's Hospital in Boston is a "one-stop shop" that streamlines the process and eliminates redundancy because clinical protocols can be standardized and uniformly applied.

"Having a dedicated preoperative clinic centralizes and standardizes the work," says Angela Bader MD, MPH, associate professor of anesthesia, Harvard Medical School, and director of the Weiner Center for Preoperative Evaluation.

Brigham has more than 40 ORs and other procedural sites that provide anesthesia services.

The clinic has a central waiting room and space for performing all assessments and laboratory work, including 16 examination rooms and a room for chart organization.

Nurse practitioners employed by the hospital and supervised by on-site anesthesiologists perform the histories and physicals as well as the anesthesiology and nursing assessments for 80 to 90 patients per day.

Many patients have complex medical conditions that warrant an intensive preop evaluation. Though Dr Bader says administrators of other hospitals have told her they don't need a preoperative clinic because of their size, she notes that even small community hospitals need a preoperative assessment program that includes all of the necessary elements.

"It's just a question of what's the most efficient, centralized way to get those elements done."

Know billing, payment systems

Understanding regulations and reimbursement policies for preop assessment is necessary to plan for the preop clinic's operational structure, Dr Bader says.

Organizing the clinic for efficient assessments is essential to the financial performance of the hospital's procedural areas. Standardizing documentation also ensures coding will be accurate. Histories and physicals (H&Ps) performed in surgeons' offices generally are not standardized, she says. They may not include all of the patients' comorbidities and may not sufficiently address medical conditions not related to the reason for the surgery.

Although reimbursement for the preop evaluation may not go directly to the clinic, she points out that the anesthesiologist, surgeon, and hospital all receive portions of the payment for the procedure.

Screening for high-risk patients

The University of Miami Health System in Florida has a preoperative clinic that covers 2 hospitals and is staffed with an anesthesiologist and internist who assess high-risk patients and supervise phone screening for all surgical patients.

"By designing the process this way, the internist is able to bill for a preoperative medical consultation, and the sicker patients benefit from seeing both an internist and an anesthesiologist," says Seema Chandra, MD, medical director of the University of Miami Health System Preoperative Assessment Center and assistant professor of clinical medicine and pediatrics. The clinic, open since February 2010, sees about 15 patients a day, with a plan to scale up to 25 to 30 a day. The hospital has 14 ORs and a related facility with 4 ORs; the combined surgical volume is about 13,000 cases.

Documenting comorbidities

High-risk patients benefit from seeing a physician preoperatively, and their comorbidities can be documented so treatments can be coded correctly for proper reimbursement, she notes. The internists and anesthesiologists have developed algorithms for the assessment, minimizing same-day testing and delays. Some of the clinic's

Process improvement

PHONE: 305-243-2196   **UPAC Preoperative Screening Form**   E-MAIL: UPAC@MED.MIAMI.EDU

1.	Do you become short of breath or develop chest pain when climbing a flight of stairs?	NO	YES
2.	Do you have high blood pressure that requires 2 or more medications to control it?	NO	YES
3.	Have you ever had heart disease, pacemaker/defibrillator, heart surgery, angioplasty or a stent placed?	NO	YES
4.	Have you ever had blood clots, stroke, carotid artery blockage, or TIA ("mini-strokes")?	NO	YES
5.	Are you currently taking blood thinners such as Coumadin (warfarin), Plavix (clopidogrel), Effient (prasugrel), etc.?	NO	YES
6.	Do you have a history of excessive bleeding following medical or dental procedures, or have you had to see a doctor due to problems with bleeding or clotting?	NO	YES
7.	Are you morbidly obese (more than 100lbs overweight)?	NO	YES
8.	Do you have asthma, chronic bronchitis, emphysema, or sleep apnea?	NO	YES
9.	In the last two years have you been on steroids like prednisone for a condition such as lupus, severe rheumatoid arthritis, chronic lung conditions, or hypopituitary condition?	NO	YES
10.	Do you have diabetes?	NO	YES
11.	Do you have kidney problems and regularly see a nephrologist (kidney specialist) or receive dialysis?	NO	YES
12.	Do you have a history of cirrhosis or chronic liver disease?	NO	YES
13.	Are you currently being treated for cancer, excluding basal cell?	NO	YES
14.	Have you or anyone in your family ever had significant complications with anesthesia other than nausea or vomiting?	NO	YES

Based on your medical history, your surgeon will determine if further medical evaluation is needed to prepare for surgery. You may be required to see a physician for evaluation and optimization of your medical condition prior to surgery, or you may be asked to complete a short phone screen with a registered nurse prior to surgery.

_____ _____ ___/___/___ _____
Patient Name (PRINT)   Signature   Date   Time

TO BE COMPLETED BY SURGEON AND/OR DESIGNEE – PLEASE FAX COMPLETED FORM TO UPAC AT 305-243-7292

SURGERY LOCATION: ☐ UMH   ☐ UMHC-SYLVESTER

☐ If responding **YES** to any questions, a preoperative consultation with a physician is recommended (select one):

☐ UPAC Physician   ☐ Primary Care Physician (PCP)   ☐ Specialist: _____

☐ If responding **NO** to all questions, patient will complete a phone screen with a registered nurse prior to surgery.

If requesting a consultation:
Based on a review of the patient's medical history and specific medical conditions outlined, a consultation with a qualified internist or specialist (as directed) is requested. This consultation is requested to minimize risks of developing complications as a result of surgery and/or anesthesia.

_____ _____ ___/___/___ _____
Surgeon Name (PRINT)   Signature   Date   Time

UHealth
UNIVERSITY OF MIAMI HEALTH SYSTEM
Preoperative Assessment Center

Preoperative Evaluation Form
Page 1 of 1 (Revised 01/29/10)

operational expenses are supported by providing the preop medical consults in addition to the preanesthesia assessments.

Presently, the surgeons perform the H&Ps, but the clinic is working with the 2 surgical sites to see if the medical consults can also be used as a surgical H&P.

The clinic's anesthesiologist already had been working at a preoperative center at the smaller of the University of Miami's hospitals and was willing to continue in that role in the combined hospital clinic. The internists who cover the center vary.

Together, the internist and anesthesiologist generate a consult that goes to the surgeon and is placed in the patient's chart. Any further testing is coordinated by the clinic.

Which patients are at high risk?

For a consult to be billable, medically necessary reasons for the consult must be documented.

A 14-point questionnaire completed in the surgeons' offices determines whether the patient needs a medical consult in the clinic. Examples of questions are: "Do you have diabetes? Have you had any cardiac procedures like a stent or pacemaker implanted?" If patients answer yes, they're eligible for a medical consultation by the preop clinic.

If the screening shows patients are at a lower risk, and the surgeon has no medical reason for referring them to the clinic, a nurse performs a telephone screening.

The same anesthesiologist who sees patients in the clinic reviews the telephone screening results. If the anesthesiologist determines that a patient needs further testing, the nurse informs the surgical coordinator, who communicates with the patient's primary care physician to order the tests. The only tests that are billable are those that are reasonable and necessary for diagnosis or treatment.

"We didn't see the value of seeing low-risk patients in the clinic because the main goal is to reduce preoperative medical risks and minimize first-case delays and same-day cancellations," says Dr Chandra. The high-risk patients, not the low-risk patients, are the ones whose cases are cancelled or delayed.

Three-tiered assessment

A 3-tiered program in the preoperative assessment service at Kettering Medical Center in Kettering, Ohio, enables surgeons to refer complex, high-risk surgical patients to a nurse practitioner for a preop H&P or to a hospitalist who will perform an H&P as well as follow the patient postoperatively. Low-risk patients have a nursing assessment.

Patients' risk is assessed using the Metabolic Equivalent Task (METs) scoring tool, a measure of a patient's physical activity level. (A METs table is available at www.americanheart.org/presenter.jhtml?identifier=3046878.)

Patients are screened when they are contacted to make their appointments. Depending on their METs score, they are scheduled for a phone or a face-to-face assessment. Surgeons can also request a face-to-face assessment for patients.

Patients are assessed in the preoperative clinic, open 5 days a week from 9 am to 7:30 pm. Kettering has 21 ORs and 2 endoscopy suites and a volume of 16,000 surgical cases a year.

The hospitalists are not employed by the hospital. They bill for their professional services, and the hospital bills for a facility component.

When the nurse practitioner performs the assessment, the hospital bills for both the nurse practitioner's services and facility services. No fee is associated with the nursing assessment, which is considered part of the preoperative evaluation.

"We have to have a minimum of 6 cases a day done by nurse practitioners to break even," says Trisha Osborn, Kettering's business manager for perioperative services.

Preoperative assessments by the nurse practitioner or physicians must be scheduled, but patients can come to the clinic any time for a nursing assessment.

Hospitalist assessments have been available for a few years. The nurse practitioner service was started about a year ago, and the "drop-in" nursing assessments began about 6 months ago. Nursing assessments also can be performed by telephone.

Day of surgery cancellations have decreased 2% since all 3 tiers of the program were initiated, says Lynn Filiatrault, RN, CNOR, clinical nurse manager.

Previously, 75% of testing and assessments were performed within 48 hours of surgery. Now most are performed 2 to 3 weeks in advance, with only 15% performed 48 hours before surgery.

Surgeons encourage program

The surgeons encouraged the creation of the preoperative assessment program, says Filiatrault. The program relieves surgeons of the assessment and ensures assessments meet regulatory requirements. The surgeons and anesthesiologists have developed a preoperative testing protocol linked to specific diagnoses and comorbidities.

Though additional reimbursement is not available for the preop screening clinic, the hospital hopes the service will pay for itself by reducing cancellations and delays, says Osborn.

The hospital found that when patients' cases had to be cancelled on the day of surgery because of incomplete testing or charts, a high percentage of those patients went somewhere else to have their surgery performed.

"For us, it became a matter of how can we get the patients through the system successfully the first time? The preoperative clinic has done that for us," says Osborn. ❖

—*Judith M. Mathias, RN, MA*

Nurse practitioner competencies used at the Brigham and Women's preoperative clinic are available from the Society for Perioperative Assessment and Quality Improvement (SPAQI) at www.spaqi.org (membership required).

References

Correll D J, Bader A M, Hull M W, et al. Value of preoperative clinic visits in identifying issues with potential impact on operating room efficiency. *Anesthesiology*. 2006;105:1254-1259.

Ferschl M B, Tung A, Sweitzer B, et al. Preoperative clinic visits reduce operating room cancellations and delays. *Anesthesiology*. 2005;103:855-859.

Harnett M J, Correll D J, Hurwitz S, et al. Improving efficiency and patient satisfaction in a tertiary teaching hospital preoperative clinic. *Anesthesiology*. 2010;112:66-72.

Yen C, Tsai M, Macario A. Preoperative evaluation clinics. *Curr Opin Anaesthesiol*. 2010;23:67-172.

This article originally appeared in OR Manager, *April 2011;27:14-17.*

Automation Ends Preop Paper Chase

Preparing patients for the day of surgery can mean chasing faxes and other documents that are easily misplaced. Missing information can lead to surgical delays and cancellations, not to mention frustrated physicians and staff.

If ever a process was ripe for automation, this is it. With the government's funding for electronic health records (EHR), the preoperative process is one area hospitals and physicians may be looking at.

One option is to harness the Internet. Preoperative documentation is submitted through a secure web portal where physicians, nurses, and other authorized users can access it easily.

OR Manager spoke with users and representatives of 3 companies that offer web-based systems for managing preoperative information.

Presurgical Care Management System

Advocate Lutheran General Hospital in Park Ridge, Illinois, has been using an automated preoperative evaluation system for about 5 years.

"We almost never cancel a case anymore because a patient hasn't been prepared appropriately preoperatively," says Mary Kay Bissing, DO, chair of anesthesia and perioperative medicine. "And we don't have to get last-minute consults, which we were doing almost daily." She estimates the software has reduced the cancellation rate from missing paperwork on the day of surgery from about 5% to near zero.

The Presurgical Care Management System was developed by David Young, MD, Advocate Lutheran General's medical director of presurgical testing. The software collects patient information, processes it into risk scores and treatment plans, and generates reports. The system is now owned by DocuSys, Inc, Atlanta (www.docusys.net). Dr Young is the company's medical director of presurgical care.

Web-based questionnaire

Patients access the automated questionnaire at home or through kiosks in surgery centers and physician offices using an identification number.

The questionnaire, developed by the Cleveland Clinic and used by the Clinic and Advocate Lutheran General, focuses mainly on pulmonary, diabetes, and cardiac issues.

Patients answer the yes or no questions phrased in layman's terms. Yes answers trigger further questions. A nurse always verifies the completed questionnaire with the patient and asks more questions if needed, Dr Young notes.

The software converts the patient's responses to medical terminology. For example, the questionnaire asks: "Do you have shortness of breath at night that requires sleeping on more than 2 pillows?" If the patient enters "yes," the program reports that the patient has "nocturnal dyspnea."

Once the information is entered and verified, the software compares the findings with the surgery the patient will have and determines the lab testing and any further evaluation needed. The system then creates different reports for the patient, surgeon, preop evaluation clinic, primary care physician, and anesthesiologist.

My Medical Files

Automation has helped end the paper chase at Christiana Care Health System, Wilmington, Delaware, which in September 2008 adopted a web-based system from My Medical Files (MMF from MMF Systems, Inc, New York City, www.mmf.com).

Before, a blizzard of faxes led to "many delays on the day of surgery and physician dissatisfaction," says Andrea Rodriguez, RN, BSN, CNOR, manager of surgical services for Christiana Care.

MMF indexes, tracks, and notifies clinicians of missing information without the involvement of hospital staff.

How it works

With MMF, patient information is faxed to a central number. The incoming faxes are received by fax services, which digitize and store the documents in a database. The documents are then made available over MMF's secure web servers in Virginia and California. Users are given a password to the MMF website.

The digitized documents then go to trained personnel in India who index patient information around the clock, making it available on the MMF website minutes after receiving it, explains Jose Barranco, MMF's vice president for market development and compliance. He says the company can provide an entire patient folder within 30 minutes of receiving a patient's documents.

None of the data actually travels to India, Barranco notes. Personnel have read-only access to the documents that remain in the secure web servers.

Missing information is tracked down by MMF

Preop automation costs

Presurgical Care Management System
DocuSys

The price is based on the hospital's annual surgical cases. The software is available as a site license or on a per-case basis. There is a one-time implementation fee and annual maintenance fee.

For a hospital with 5,000 cases a year, the base one-time license fee is about $80,000 plus implementation services and an annual maintenance fee of $15,000.

For a surgical center with 2,000 cases per year, the base one-time license fee is about $25,000 plus implementation and an annual maintenance fee of $5,000.

Alternatively, the system is offered for a per-patient fee of $2.50 to $6.50, depending on volumes and configuration.

—*www.docusys.net*

My Medical File
MMF Systems

Fees are based on the number of procedures a facility performs.

For indexing 10,000 cases a year, MMF charges $4,000 a month. Include in the request for proposal the number of representatives the company will provide for training and for how long, advises Andrea Rodriguez, RN, BSN, CNOR, of Christiana Care, Wilmington, Delaware, which uses MMF.

—*www.mmf.com*

One Medical Passport
Medical Web Technologies

Pricing varies based on the configuration, modules purchased, and surgical volume.

A community hospital with a standard configuration, for example, could expect to pay about $1,000 to $2,000 per month.

—*www.onemedicalpassport.com*

---

staff based in Panama (who speak fluent English), who phone surgeons' offices.

Patients' folders can be accessed by Christiana Care clinicians and office staff. Patients do not have access to the file.

"I can't tell you how much the tracking service has changed the quality of life at the points of service," says Rodriguez.

Eliminating the paper shuffle

The day before surgery, the OR staff prints out a hard copy of the patient's folder.

"We still need a hard copy of the patient's chart. But we have eliminated 60,000 pieces of paper we were shuffling each month," says Rodriguez, noting physician satisfaction with MMF is high.

Anesthesia providers print out the patient's information because the anesthesia department does not have an automated information system yet. The goal is to go paperless.

One Medical Passport

One Medical Passport (Medical Web Technologies, Scituate, Massachusetts) is a different approach, giving patients a free portable health record. Individuals can set up a "medical passport" on the company's website (www.onemedicalpassport.com) and keep it for their records.

"Patients have a tremendous interest in creating a personal health record, and One Medical Passport is a great tool for doing this. There is no charge to patients," says Stephen Punzak, MD, an anesthesiologist who is the company's founder and CEO.

Health care facilities and physician offices pay a fee to access a patient's One Medical Passport information, with the patient's permission.

Geared for first-time users

Typically, patients find out about One Medical Passport when they schedule surgery with a hospital or surgeon who uses the system. The surgeon gives the patient a card with the surgery date, type of surgery, and how to access the website. The patient logs on at home, creates a user name and password, and fills out the online questionnaire. Patients cannot skip questions and can review the information before it is submitted.

"The system is geared for people who have never used it before and for those with limited computer experience," says Dan Short, Medical Web Technologies's vice president of sales.

The completed passport data is stored in the company's secure storage facility and can be downloaded by any provider a patient has granted access to. The information either is displayed in a report format that can be printed or in an electronic format that can be interfaced.

Power of the passport

The power of the One Medical Passport technology is not only in the data collection but also in what it does with the data, Dr Punzak says. Rather than simply printing out the patient's information, the system routes the information to the clinician who needs it.

An Assessment Checklist module lists tasks and forms that need to be completed for each patient. As information comes in, the system automatically takes the task off the list. An audit trail shows who indicated the task was completed and when.

A document manager module automatically scans documents, alerts the facility the documents have been submitted, and automatically alerts the surgeon's office if documentation is missing.

More accurate information

A surgery center that has used One Medical Passport for about a year finds the system has improved the accuracy of patient information.

Patients can fill out the online questionnaire from their homes in a relaxed manner, which helps ensure the information is correct and complete, says Gina Espenschied, RN, BSN, CNOR, administrator of The Surgery Center at Brinton Lake, Glen Mills, Pennsylvania, which performs about 500 to 600 cases a month.

"In the past, when preoperative nurses called patients, they often caught them in the car or at work with little time to focus on the questions," she says. As a result, the information sometimes wasn't complete or differed from what the patient gave on the day of surgery.

Espenschied says the document manager module has decreased surgery cancellations caused by missing paperwork by nearly 15%. About 70% of patients complete the Passport compared to 20% when the program was introduced. ❖

— *Judith M. Mathias, RN, MA*

This article originally appeared in OR Manager, *June 2009;25:11-12,14.*

VII. Scheduling

Fine-Tuning the Block Schedule? Now Could Be the Right Time

If you want to fine-tune the block schedule, now may be the time. A silver lining of the recession is that surgeons and staff may be more accepting of changes to the schedule than they might be otherwise.

With the decline in elective surgery from the economic downturn, surgeons are less able to leverage one hospital against another.

In all, by the end of March 2009, 59% of hospitals were seeing a moderate or significant decrease in elective procedures, the American Hospital Association reports.

"This is allowing hospitals to make changes that are more politically challenging," observes William Mazzei, MD, medical director of perioperative services and clinical professor of anesthesiology at the University of California, San Diego.

"What is important to surgeons is good use of their time at one facility rather than playing one facility against another. They don't have the business to do that any more."

Facilities may be able to enforce stricter rules to improve OR utilization, he says. With more OR time available, they may be able to encourage surgeons to stay at the facility longer than they might have in ordinary times.

For example, if the OR has allowed some surgeons to have half-day blocks, which is not optimal for utilization, it may be easier to make these full-day blocks.

If the surgeons object, the facility might respond by saying it will convert these blocks to open time into which anyone can schedule cases. In this environment, most surgeons will accept the change, says Dr Mazzei, who is also with Surgical Directions LLC, Chicago-based consultants.

It may also be easier to match staffing more closely to the surgical schedule, he notes. In a down economy, staff may be more accepting of scheduling changes.

The business of blocks

With fewer cases, ORs need to pay close attention to how surgeons' block time is affecting their business, comments Jerry Ippolito, MBA, MHSA, of consultants OR Efficiencies LLC, Naples, Florida.

When a surgeon asks for block time, he suggests the question should be: "What are you going to bring us?" How will the surgeon's cases benefit the hospital? He advises posing the same question to surgeons who already have block time.

The block time analysis should include not only how much of their block time surgeons are using but also the contribution margin of their cases. (Contribution margin = revenue − variable costs, such as implants and specialty staffing). The contribution margin should be calculated before indirect costs are allocated and should include revenue and expenses for the surgeon's patients hospitalwide, not just for the OR, he adds.

The literature includes a number of studies on OR time allocation, including use of contribution margin.

Good governance

Nothing is more important to effective block scheduling than strong, active leadership, these experts say. The block scheduling system must be governed by policies and procedures endorsed by the medical staff and enforced by the OR's governing body. Policies must be transparent.

"The system must be scrupulously fair. If there is any favoritism, the surgeons will sniff it out, and it will never work," stresses Tom Blasco, MD, MS, an anesthesiologist and intensivist at Advocate Lutheran General Hospital, Park Ridge, Illinois, and a consultant with Surgical Directions LLC.

The OR governing body must be committed to ongoing measurement and evaluation, Ippolito adds. "Many organizations allocate block time to a surgeon and never look at it again, whether the surgeon uses it or not."

When blocks are poorly managed, surgeons have bad experiences and may end up rejecting block scheduling all together. (For more on OR governance, see the July 2008 OR Manager.)

Communication is a corollary

Communicating with surgeons about their blocks is essential in managing the block schedule, says Stephanie Davis, RN, MS, CNOR, assistant vice president, surgical services for the HCA Clinical Services Group of HCA Inc, the national health care company based in Nashville, Tennessee.

The surgeon's office often schedules the cases. The office may be scheduling some cases outside the block because these other times are more convenient, she notes.

"If we are not transparent with surgeons about their utilization, they may not know they are not meeting the target. They may volunteer on their own to adjust their block," she says.

Open communication is also part of customer service.

"If you have a good relationship with your surgeons, they will trust you to manage blocks fairly," says Davis, who has assembled a block scheduling toolkit for HCA Inc's 165 hospitals (related article, p 80).

Starting a conversation

Good relationships make it easier to start a conversation if a surgeon's block utilization is not what is expected. Davis says that when she was a perioperative director, she talked to the surgeons about low utilization as soon as she found out.

She might say, for example, "Dr Smith, I hope you got your letter about block utilization. Did you realize you were only running about 35%? Do you want to move your block to a different day? What can I do to help you get your utilization where it needs to be?"

Efforts to manage the block schedule can be worth it because everyone benefits, Dr Mazzei observes.

"The workday is more enjoyable for physicians and staff alike in hospitals that have completely full blocks, do lots of cases during the day, and have limited overtime and limited nights and weekends," he says. "They find this is a win-win situation." That may not be obvious to people in systems that have had the same underutilized block times for 20 years, he adds. Today's environment may create the opportunity to change that situation. ❖

—Pat Patterson

References

Mclntosh C, Dexter F, Epstein R H. Impact of service-specific staffing, case scheduling, turnovers, and first-case starts on anesthesia group and operating room productivity: A tutorial using data from an Australian hospital. *Anesth Analg.* 2006;103:1499-1516.

Patterson P. A few simple rules for managing block time in the operating room. *OR Manager.* 2004; 20(11):1, 9-12.

Patterson P. Is your OR's governing structure up to today's intense demands? *OR Manager.* 2008;24(7):1, 6-7.

Wachter R E, Dexter F. Tactical increases in operating room block time for capacity planning should not be based on utilization. *Anesth Analg,* 2008:106:215-226.

This article originally appeared in OR Manager, *July 2009;25:1,8,12.*

A Toolkit for Managing Block Scheduling

HCA Inc, the national health care company, has developed a block scheduling toolkit for its 165 hospitals. The toolkit includes decision points, algorithms for managing blocks, and sample policies.

Here are HCA Inc's 10 decision points for block scheduling.

1. Is this the right time for block scheduling?

About 75% to 80% of HCA Inc's hospitals use block scheduling, estimates Stephanie Davis, RN, MS, CNOR, assistant vice president, surgical services for the HCA Clinical Services Group, Nashville, Tennessee, who developed the toolkit.

If an OR isn't using block scheduling, she suggests asking: "What are the reasons for not offering this service? Are those reasons still valid in today's environment?"

Not every OR decides to use block allocations. "If you don't have a lot of volume and are trying to get every case you can, you might not want to rock the boat with the medical staff," she notes.

In some parts of the country, "surgeons are really anti-block," says Jerry Ippolito, MBA, MHSA, director of perioperative services and pain management business development, Southeast Anesthesiology Consultants, Charlotte, NC.

That can happen if they have had a bad experience. To some, block scheduling means "preferential treatment." Surgeons may be more receptive to another term, such as "reserved time," he suggests.

An OR schedule with all open time has its own problems, he adds. Open time favors surgeons who perform mostly elective cases, such as ENT and ophthalmology, and can schedule far in advance.

Even in an OR with all open time, surgeons tend to establish patterns that are, in effect, like block time.

Leaders may have success getting the surgeons to accept block scheduling if they show them data demonstrating that their cases already fall into regular patterns, he suggests.

How much time should be blocked? Typically, 55% to 80%, though how much open time to offer depends on the situation, Ippolito says. A high-volume trauma center can't allocate as much time as an OR with a more predictable caseload. How much time to leave open is also a strategic issue. A more mature setting may have 80% to 85% of its time blocked, while a facility trying to attract new surgeons will want more open time available.

2. Does your block scheduling policy include key elements?

Davis suggests key elements of the policy should include:

- A block utilization rate is calculated monthly and reported to each surgeon quarterly. The toolkit recommends a block utilization rate of 70%. But there is no hard-and-fast rule, Davis says.

"It's up to our facilities to set the level they think is appropriate." Davis says monitoring of blocks requires discernment: "Your OR governance team has to look at each situation and be able to back up its decisions with facts."

(From a scientific point of view, adjusting blocks according to utilization isn't the best choice, notes a leading researcher, Franklin Dexter, MD, PhD. See related article, p 82.)

- Automatic block release times are stated and enforced consistently for all surgeons. In a general OR with a lot of specialties, a 72-hour release is appropriate, Davis says. "Some will argue 48 hours is better; others will argue 1 week. You have to decide with your group what fits." One option is release times by specialty (sidebar).

- The policy states that if a surgeon notifies the OR in advance to release block time, unused time will not count against the surgeon in the block utilization report. Advance notice allows other procedures to be booked into the unused time.

3. Is there a physician champion?

Blocks are best managed by an executive committee made up of the OR director, the administrator responsible for surgery, the chief of surgery, and the chief of anesthesia.

"Everyone on the committee has a vested interest in making block scheduling work," Davis notes.

The physician champion helps to monitor and enforce the block schedule and communicate with the surgeons.

"Communication goes over better if the surgeon receives it from a peer," she notes.

The physician champion, with the OR director, should be willing to sign letters to the surgeons informing them of their block utilization.

4. Is there a grace period?

The block scheduling policy allows surgeons a 3-month grace period to improve their block utilization once informed of their utilization rates, the toolkit advises.

"Our plan is to inform surgeons of their block utilization once a quarter but to tell them we will wait one more quarter before doing anything to their block to allow for variances," Davis says.

5. How is the utilization rate communicated?

"It's important to communicate with every surgeon. If they have a block, you communicate with them once a quarter, regardless of their utilization," Davis says.

The toolkit recommends a tiered approach to communication. For example:

- A letter of congratulation is sent to surgeons with a block utilization rate of 70% or greater.
- Surgeons with utilization of 70% to 50% are informed they have not met the threshold and asked to decrease the time blocked or to consider changing their day or time to improve usage.
- Surgeons whose utilization falls below 50% are informed they are well below the threshold, and if they do not bring their utilization to 70% or above by the end of the next quarter, they will lose the privilege of having a block.

6. Are at least 1 or 2 ORs reserved for first-come, first-served booking?

"Having open rooms allows new surgeons to book occasional cases in your OR and allows for recruitment of new business," Davis notes.

7. Do you have 1 OR for add-ons, emergencies, and flip-flopping of cases?

"In small ORs, this might not be possible, but in medium to large ORs, it is effective," Davis says.

Open rooms provide flexibility to move cases and add cases. There may be exceptions for facilities such as eye centers where routines are well established. The rule is not rigid; the point is to have flexibility. Providing an add-on room for urgent and emergent cases enabled St John's Regional Health Center, a regional trauma center in Springfield, Missouri, to increase its surgical volume by 5%, increase surgeon revenue by 4.6%, reduce the need for ORs after 3 pm, and reduce overtime. The project was part of an effort to smooth patient flow throughout the hospital. (See November 2003 and January 2005 OR Manager.)

Suggested block release times

Burn service (inpatient)	1 day
Cardiac	1 day
General surgery	7 days
Gynecology	7 days
Head and neck	7 days
Neurosurgery	4 days
Ophthalmology	7 days
Orthopedics (joint)	14 days
Orthopedics (spine)	3 days
Pediatrics	7 days
Plastic (cosmetic)	14 days
Radiology	3 days
Vascular	2 days
Thoracic	3 days

Source: William J. Mazzei, MD; Tom Blasco, MD. OR Manager. 2004;20(11):1, 9-12.

8. Is the schedule accurate?

Are your OR analyst and schedulers making sure the schedule is accurate so utilization reports will reflect accurately each surgeon's block use? Accurate data is critical when reporting block utilization to surgeons.

9. Are you willing to enforce the block scheduling policy fairly?

Effective block scheduling requires maintenance and enforcement of rules, Davis says. The HCA Inc toolkit provides a sample policy for block scheduling.

10. Will the administration support the block scheduling policy?

Effective block scheduling always comes back to good governance. The administration must support the surgical executive committee that reviews the block allocations and not overturn their decisions. ❖

References

Hospital moves to smooth surgery schedule. *OR Manager.* 2003; 19(11):11.

Questions managers ask about patient flow. *OR Manager.* 2005; 21(1):20-21.

Smoothing OR schedule can ease capacity crunches, researchers say. *OR Manager.* 2003;19(11):1, 9-10.

This article originally appeared in OR Manager, *July 2009;25:9-10.*

The Research on OR Time Allocation

What criteria should be used to make decisions about adjusting block time? Traditionally, OR committees have used surgeons' utilization of blocks. But OR utilization isn't the best way to make this decision, the research shows.

The method to use depends on why block time is being adjusted, notes Franklin Dexter, MD, PhD: Are blocks being adjusted for operational reasons; that is, to match staffing to the existing OR workload? Or are blocks being adjusted for tactical reasons, such as to provide more convenient access to OR time for some surgeons?

Consider these scenarios:

Scenario 1: Tactical decision

A group of neurosurgeons has 91% utilization of their block time. They're recruiting a new spine surgeon and need more OR time.

Dr Jenkins, a vascular surgeon, has 60% utilization of his block. It seems that he could use less time.

Should the OR committee take some of Dr Jenkins's block time and give it to the neurosurgeons? This is a tactical decision.

Scenario 2: Operational decision

The neuro service has a block allocation of 3 ORs on Mondays from 7:15 am to 3:30 pm. They have little underutilized time and often have overutilized time (ie, run late). How many nursing staff should be assigned for 8 hours and how many for 10 hours? This is an operational decision.

Tactical decisions

For tactical decisions like Scenario 1, decisions increasingly are being made at least partly to meet financial goals, Dr Dexter says. The OR committee might, for example, look at the contribution margin for spinal surgery to decide if giving the neurosurgeons more block time would help the hospital financially. (Contribution margin = revenue − variable costs.) More spinal surgery might or might not be a good idea, depending on the implant costs and the reimbursement.

Tactical decisions also include strategic issues. Dr Dexter says "revenue" should be considered from a long-term perspective and should include not only reimbursement but also the intangible value of adding more cases in a focused strategic area. For example, executives decide your hospital is going to be a regional pediatric center. Of course, you will give your pediatric surgeon a great deal of block time, the cost and reimbursement issues aside. In this case, each additional pediatric patient has an intangible value, known in economics as utility, Dr Dexter explains.

Utilization not best choice for tactical decisions

Utilization is not the best choice for making tactical decisions on block time, Dr Dexter says, citing 5 reasons from the literature:

1. Utilization does not help to reduce patient waiting times, which is usually a goal of patients as well as clinicians and administrators.

2. Utilization is poorly related to contribution margin. A surgeon or service with high utilization can still lose the hospital money if reimbursement for these cases doesn't cover costs.

3. Efforts to increase utilization can actually reduce margins. For example, the hospital signs an insurance contract hoping to increase surgical volume, but not many of the patients have surgery, and the contracted rates are too low to cover costs.

4. Utilization is poorly related to variable costs. Surgeons with equal utilizations can have different variable costs. For example, 2 surgeons have 70% block utilization. The first surgeon performs outpatient breast surgery, which has low variable costs per OR hour. The second surgeon performs joint replacements, which have high variable costs per OR hour.

5. For surgeons with low utilization, it is questionable whether utilization can be estimated sufficiently precisely for this purpose. A 2003 study found, for example, that if during 1 quarter, Surgeon 1 had a block utilization of 65%, and Surgeon 2 had a block utilization of 80%, statistically, the difference may be due to random chance. For surgeons with low utilization, the study found it would take more than 10 years of data to measure block utilization accurately enough to be of practical value in making block-time decisions.

Operational decisions

Operational decisions should be made to improve OR efficiency, according to research findings. For this purpose, OR efficiency is defined as a balance between underutilized and overutilized OR time. If time is underutilized, revenue isn't coming in while the OR is incurring labor costs.

Overutilized time means clinicians have to work late, which is a dissatisfier and can be costly if overtime is needed.

Achieving OR efficiency involves matching the staffing allocation as closely as possible to the existing workload.

In Scenario 2, depending on the details of the neuro service workload, a decision based on OR efficiency might be to increase the neuro service's OR allocation (or block) from 7:15 am to 6 pm in 2 of the 3 ORs. The anesthesia providers and nurses gain by having more predictable work hours (ie, fewer overutilized hours).

The purpose of this block adjustment is not to encourage more neurosurgery because the neurosurgeons are already getting their cases on the schedule. Rather, the purpose is to achieve a better balance between underutilized and overutilized time.

"Generally, what surgeons care about are tactical decisions: 'How can I grow my practice?'" Dr Dexter says. "What anesthesiologists and nurses generally care about are decisions on the day of surgery: 'Will I finish on time?'" ❖

More information on Dr Dexter's research and consulting is at www.FranklinDexter.net

References

Dexter F, Blake J T, Penning D H, et al. Use of linear programming to estimate impact of changes in a hospital's operating room time allocation on perioperative variable costs. *Anesthesiology*. March 2002;96:718-724.

Dexter F, Macario A, Traub R D, et al. Operating room utilization alone is not an accurate metric for the allocation of operating room block time to individual surgeons with low caseloads. *Anesthesiology*. May 2003;98: 1243-1249.

McIntosh C, Dexter F, Epstein R H. Impact of service-specific staffing, case scheduling, turnovers, and first-case starts on anesthesia group and operating room productivity: A tutorial using data from an Australian hospital. *Anesth Analg*. 2006;103:1499-1516.

O'Neill L, Dexter F. Tactical increases in operating room block time based on financial data and market growth estimates from data envelopment analysis. *Anesth Analg*. 2007;104:355-368.

Wachter R E, Dexter F. Tactical increases in operating room block time for capacity planning should not be based on utilization. *Anesth Analg*. 2008;106:215-226.

This article originally appeared in OR Manager, *July 2009;25:11-12.*

Effective Block Scheduling Rests on Fair Policies, Active Management

Performing more cases with the same OR capacity and personnel—and having more satisfied surgeons, anesthesia providers, and staff. That may sound like utopia, but there is a way to make it happen. The answer is a well-run block scheduling program. The need to manage OR time effectively is increasingly important as hospitals brace for lower reimbursement as part of health care reform. Hospital leaders will be looking to surgery as one way to maximize revenue while reducing costs.

If your block scheduling program could use a tune-up, a set of guidelines developed by a veteran perioperative medical director can help improve OR utilization, generate more revenue, and increase satisfaction.

William Mazzei, MD, has worked with hospitals on OR-related issues for nearly 25 years. He is clinical professor of anesthesiology and was medical director of perioperative services at the University of California, San Diego, for 20 years. He is also a founder of the American Association of Clinical Directors (originally the Association of Anesthesia Clinical Directors) and one author of the procedural times glossary.

(See the related article on p 82 for the research perspective on managing block allocations, which includes examining the financial implications of block time decisions.)

Guiding principles

Effective block scheduling, Dr Mazzei says, rests on a few principles. The program:

- is guided by policies that are transparent, developed by consensus, and perceived as fair
- is actively managed by a collaborative team of leaders from surgery, nursing, anesthesia, and the hospital administration
- allows surgeons access to the OR schedule while achieving high utilization.

"Management of blocks must be done collaboratively," Dr Mazzei says. "It must consider everyone's perspective so problems can be acknowledged and discussed."

Guidelines for blocks

The guidelines he advocates govern who has block time, the balance between block and open time, and the rules for scheduling.

Who can have a block?

Blocks can be assigned to individual surgeons, groups, or services. "It doesn't matter as long as the people assigned the block understand that they are responsible for filling it," Dr Mazzei says.

Insist on 8-hour blocks

In general, blocks should be 8 hours long or an entire shift. "This is perhaps the most important guideline for efficiency and satisfaction," he says.

Benefits of 8-hour blocks include:

- minimizing gaps during the day and use of overtime
- increasing surgical volume because surgeons know they need to maintain utilization to keep their block time.
- allowing the use of specialty teams.

The 8-hour blocks make good use of surgeons' times, Dr Mazzei says, though they may need to be convinced of that initially.

"If a surgeon tends to operate for 8 hours every Monday, then having a block is the most efficient use of his or her time," he contends. "It also allows facilities to plan and have the right staff available."

Apply the 80-20 rule

In block scheduling, the 80-20 rule means:

- Up to 80% of available rooms can be blocked in a system that is working well.
- The remaining 20% of rooms are not blocked and are designated as open or urgent/emergent rooms. For centers with fewer than 10 ORs, it is generally better that at least 2 ORs remain as open rooms.

Having open rooms ensures that surgeons who don't have block time or who have little block time can get on the schedule in a reasonable time.

Vary release times by specialty

Release times for blocks, also called expiration times, are another way to provide open time and serve as an incentive for surgeons to use their blocks. Typically, release times are geared to how far in advance each specialty schedules its elective cases (chart). Alternatively, some facilities

Suggested release time guidelines

Specialty	Days*	Specialty	Days*
Cardiac	5 pm previous business day	Orthopedics	7
General surgery	3-7	Orthopedics (spine)	3
Gynecology	7	Plastic (cosmetic)	7
Head and neck	7	Vascular surgery	3
Neurosurgery	3	Urology	7
Neurosurgery (spine)	3	Ophthalmology	7

No release time if block utilization consistently exceeds 85%. *Days refer to calendar dates.

use a standard 5-day release time.

This rule has several corollaries:

Corollary 1

Surgeons may release blocks for open use only with a 30-day notice. This is far enough in advance to allow others to access the block and prevents surgeons from releasing unused time at the last minute to avoid having it count against their utilization.

Corollary 2

Surgeons cannot schedule outside their block on days they have a block. "That prevents them from using the open room first and then switching those cases to the block at the last minute if their block isn't filled," he says.

Corollary 3

Surgeons cannot release a portion of their block. For example, if an 8-hour block has only 6 hours of cases, the surgeon can't simply release the remaining 2 hours. "Release at the last minute doesn't allow anyone else access to that time," he explains. "It games the system because it allows someone to adapt their block to their utilization after the fact."

Corollary 4

Any cases a surgeon performs on his or her block day count toward the surgeon's utilization statistics, even if the case is scheduled in the block after the time has been released.

Corollary 5

Don't artificially constrict a surgeon's block. For instance, a surgeon with an 8-hour block has 6 hours of cases and wants to book a 2½ hour case. Or a surgeon wants to work for 10 hours every Tuesday.

"By allowing that, you greatly reduce dissatisfaction," he says. "You also greatly reduce 'creative scheduling' where someone tells you a case is going to take 1 hour when you know it is really going to take 3 hours.

"It's better to say to a surgeon that on any day you have a block, you can book it for as long as you want. That is a major surgeon satisfier. This is something they see as positive at the same time you are reducing other means of access."

Making the case for 8-hour blocks

Moving to 8-hour blocks may be a tough sell initially with surgeons. But once they make the change, "they are much happier," Dr Mazzei says, adding that with health care reform, hospitals will find shorter blocks financially unsustainable because too much time is unused.

Surgeons who have shorter blocks typically like to operate in the morning, go to their office in the afternoon, and come back to operate late in the day. In contrast, with an 8-hour block, a surgeon can plan to spend the whole day in the OR and schedule office visits for other days.

"Surgeons who have converted to an 8-hour block will tell you that on the day they are in the OR, their day is less stressful because they don't have to worry about being in the office. They get more done, and they tend to finish earlier because their day is more efficient," he says. "Similarly, the days they are in the office go better because they are not worried about going to the OR. They see more patients and get more done."

How do you make the case? Dr Mazzei suggests having a surgeon who already has switched to 8-hour blocks talk to the others. This may mean scheduling a call or visit with a surgeon from outside the facility.

Open rooms

A few rules govern use of the open rooms available each day.

- Open rooms are first-come, first-served. The only exception is that a surgeon cannot use them on a day he or she already has block time.
- Open rooms are available until 12 noon on the day before surgery. Then they are assigned at the discretion of the OR medical and nursing directors to streamline the schedule.

Steps for introducing new block scheduling rules

1. Review the current policies for scheduling cases and managing the block schedule. Determine what the new policies should be.
2. Propose new policies and gain consensus of the Surgical Services Executive Committee.
3. Hold a retreat for the medical staff to introduce the proposed changes to all of the surgeons. It helps if the retreat is held on a weekend in a social atmosphere, which tends to encourage more collegiality. "When you meet with all of the surgeons, you will hear feedback you didn't hear before. That lets you make changes," says William Mazzei, MD.
4. After the retreat, revise the policies based on the feedback and publish the final policies.
5. Conduct a final meeting to present the policies that is open to all surgical services medical staff. Explain these are the final policies and invite any remaining comments. State when the policies will be implemented.
6. Present the new guidelines to the surgeons, perioperative staff, and surgeons' office managers. Meet with all surgeons' offices over the next few months. Ask: Do they understand the new rules? Have you missed anything? Is there anything the hospital can do to help them with scheduling?
7. Implement the new policies with sufficient lead time to avoid disturbing the existing schedule. That generally takes about 2 months, providing time to meet with the surgeons' offices before the implementation date.

- Except for the first case, other starts in open rooms may be delayed by up to 2 hours to accommodate earlier-starting cases.

This rule helps to address the problem of surgeons who don't want to operate before 9 am or so, leaving the 7:30 am time open. The solution is a bumping policy that allows an early surgeon to bump someone who is later. For example, a surgeon has a 9 am case in the open room, and another surgeon wants to book a 2-hour case. That case can go at 7:30 am with the following caveats:

- The case can't be booked less than 2 days in advance, allowing the later surgeon who is bumped enough time to rearrange his or her schedule.
- The later surgeon must be given the "first right of refusal." That is, the later surgeon must be asked if he or she can move up his or her case to 7:30 am. If the surgeon cannot, the schedulers may delay the later surgeon's start time by up to 2 hours.

Managing block time

Once you introduce these rules, how do you monitor them and make sure the system runs smoothly? That requires active management by a collaborative team, Dr Mazzei says.

Governance structure

He advocates a surgical services executive committee, similar to a board of directors for the OR. The committee is composed primarily of surgeons and includes leaders from nursing, anesthesia, and the hospital administration. One charge of the committee is to implement, monitor, and manage the block scheduling system.

It's best if a hospital administrator, ideally the CEO, is present at each meeting.

"When the CEO attends regularly, you can make the most progress because people actually believe something will happen," he says.

"It also helps ensure someone can't go around the committee and talk to the CEO because the CEO is there."(For more on OR governance, see the June 2010 OR Manager.)

Monitoring block utilization

Blocks are monitored monthly, with regular feedback to surgeons, using adjusted utilization, which includes turnover time. For example, a surgeon with an 8-hour block who starts at 7:30 am and finishes at 12:30 pm would have 5 hours of utilization, or 62.5%.

At least 75% utilization is expected for a surgeon to retain all the block time. Why 75%?

He explains: If a surgeon has an 8-hour block but uses 5½ hours, the utilization is 68.5%, leaving 2½ hours a day unused. Requiring 75% utilization encourages the surgeon to schedule an extra case to keep block time. "Invariably, when we implement this guideline, we find many services will schedule an additional case out of the worry they will lose their block."

More cases, happier personnel

ORs that implement and actively manage a block scheduling system using these guidelines see surgeon satisfaction increase, he says, because even though rules restrict use of blocks, open time increases, and surgeons can run cases past the end of their blocks.

"Surgeons think access to the OR has improved, and thus, their satisfaction has improved."

The hospital benefits because surgeons increase their volume to retain their blocks, bringing in more revenue. Nurse managers and staff are happier because the schedule is more predictable, teams can be assigned to work with surgeons who have all-day blocks, and more cases are completed during prime day-time hours. ❖

Dr Mazzei credits the research of Franklin Dexter, MD, PhD, for informing his work on block scheduling.

This article originally appeared in OR Manager, *July 2010;26:1,6-8,10.*

Reference

AACD glossary of times used for scheduling and monitoring of diagnostic and therapeutic procedures. *Perioperative Standards and Recommended Practices.* Denver CO: AORN, 2010.

For Urgent and Emergent Cases, Which One Goes to the OR First?

When several patients needing urgent or emergent surgery arrive at a hospital simultaneously, who decides which case goes to the OR first? For true emergencies, the decision is generally straightforward, with the patient rushed into the first available room. But in many other situations, the decision is not as clear: Should the patient with an open fracture go first? Should it be the patient with an ectopic pregnancy or perhaps the patient with an intestinal obstruction? Does the most senior surgeon get the first available OR slot? Should the decision be made on the basis of first-come, first-served? Or maybe the most assertive surgeon gets his or her case in first?

Often, the decision falls to the anesthesiologist of the day in the OR. But no matter who makes the decision, the competition between surgeons and arguments with anesthesiologists cause frustration. At times, patients end up waiting for surgery longer than is clinically optimal.

Ideally, the decision should be based on an objective measure that reflects the clinical needs of the patient and gives surgeons, anesthesiologists, and OR staff a predictable and fair system for prioritizing cases.

Using a classification system for urgent surgery, such as the one described in this article, also is the first step toward improving the flow of patients through the organization. Because the OR is the hub of inpatient flow, streamlining flow through the OR will also improve flow through the organization.

A classification system

Wellstar Kennestone Hospital, a 600-bed hospital in Marietta, Georgia, working with Press Ganey, developed an innovative approach to this problem. As part of an initiative to improve patient flow through the OR, the surgical services committee, composed of respected surgeons and anesthesiologists representing different services, developed criteria for classifying all emergent and urgent cases based on the medical needs of the patient. The classification system was then used to determine the order in which cases were taken into the OR. It created a system that was fair, predictable, and based on clinically defined criteria. The clinical urgency system was used with other patient flow improvement initiatives, including designating separate ORs for these add-on cases.

Before the classification system was developed, there were no time limits for urgent/emergent cases at scheduling, and add-on cases were taken in the order posted unless they were true life- or limb-threatening emergencies.

Urgent categories and case examples

Category	Definition	Waiting time limit	Examples
A	Acute life-and-death emergencies	30–60 minutes	Massive bleeding and airway emergencies
B	Emergent but not immediately life threatening	< 2 hours	Acute spinal cord compression, bladder rupture, ectopic pregnancy
C	Urgent cases	< 4 hours	Asymptomatic foreign body, appendicitis with sepsis/rapid progression, biliary obstruction, open fracture
D	Semi-urgent cases	< 8 hours	Appendicitis, closed reduction of fracture, empyema
E	Nonurgent cases	< 24 hours	Facial nerve decompression, femoral neck fractures, mastoidectomy

Main operating room: Compliance with waiting time limits for urgent/emergent cases

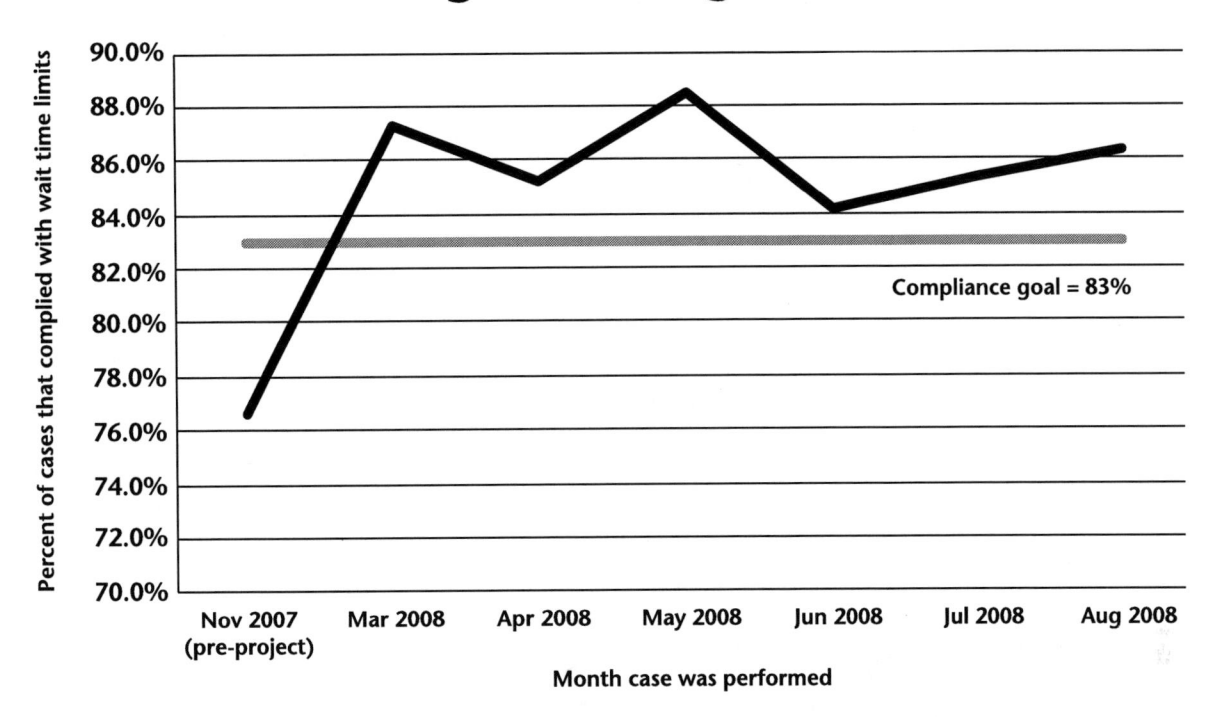

[Line chart showing Percent of cases that complied with wait time limits by Month case was performed. Nov 2007 (pre-project): ~76.5%; Mar 2008: ~87.3%; Apr 2008: ~85.3%; May 2008: ~88.7%; Jun 2008: ~84.3%; Jul 2008: ~85.7%; Aug 2008: ~86.5%. Horizontal line indicates Compliance goal = 83%.]

Case categories

The surgical services committee decided to use 5 categories to classify urgent and emergent cases. Time limits were set for each category, defining the maximum time that should pass between when a case was posted and when the patient was taken into the OR (sidebar). Each specialty reviewed its common procedures and placed them in the category in which they would most commonly fall.

How the classifications work

Once the categories were developed and accepted by the surgeons, they began to use them to specify the urgency of add-on cases as they posted them. The system works in the following way:

When a surgeon posts a case, he or she classifies it using the A-E categories based on the needs of the patient. The appropriateness of the classification is never questioned at the time the case is posted but may be reviewed by the committee retrospectively. The order in which add-on urgent/emergent cases are then scheduled into the OR is based on the urgency of the case and the amount of time since the case was posted. If 2 cases within the same category arrive close together, they are taken first-come, first-served. As time passes and the time limit approaches, cases are escalated to the highest category to ensure the patient is taken care of in the appropriate time frame.

The surgeon booking the case is responsible for categorizing the case based on knowledge of the clinical needs of the patient. For example, a surgeon can call an appendicitis case a 'B' case if he thinks the patient's condition warrants surgery within 2 hours, even though most appendicitis cases are usually considered to be in the D (within 8 hours) category. At the time of booking, no one can question the surgeon on this decision because it is assumed he or she is the one with the most accurate assessment of the situation.

Monitoring compliance

Like any system, this one can be manipulated, and oversight is necessary to maintain consistency and monitor compliance with the urgency categories. At WellStar Kennestone Hospital, the surgical services committee took on this role. Each month, the committee reviewed all 'A' cases and any other cases where the appropriateness of the urgency classification was questioned by another surgeon, an anesthesiologist, or surgical staff. If further review appeared necessary, a member of the committee talked with the surgeon in question. If systematic or frequent problems occurred, the surgeon would be asked to appear before the committee to discuss the cases. This peer review system is critical to maintain accurate categorization and to avoid gaming of the system. The review can also lead to revisions to the category guidelines over time.

Waiting times decline

With the implementation of this approach to scheduling urgent/emergent cases, waiting

Improving OR Performance The OR Management Series

times for these cases declined by 18% overall. For urgent and semi-urgent cases—types of cases that typically get delayed—the decreases in waiting time were even more dramatic, with waiting times decreasing 77% for C cases (maximum wait 4 hours) and 33% for D cases (maximum wait 8 hours). In addition, E (nonurgent same day) cases no longer got pushed into nighttime hours (11 pm to 7 am) because there was more time during the day to get these cases completed. The number of staff needed at night was reduced because the staff had to care only for more urgent cases.

The surgeons were pleased that their patients were getting into the OR more quickly. Surgeons, anesthesiologists, and OR staff appreciated the transparency of the system. "Since we are able to get critical cases done more quickly," said an anesthesiologist, "we end up with less of a backlog during the day and no longer find ourselves doing hip fractures at midnight."

To determine the capacity necessary to accommodate add-on cases, a queuing analysis was done to determine how much staffed capacity was needed for these cases. The queuing analysis was key to ensuring that the urgent/emergent cases would have appropriate access to the OR, but elective cases could proceed without bumping or delays. This was accomplished without building new OR space.

The block schedule was revised to minimize gaps during the day and was built based on utilization and the patient's destination unit, reducing peaks and valleys in the day-to-day surgical schedule.

Success factors

The use of a consistent clinically based system for prioritizing add-on cases can solve the difficult problem of "who gets in first." These features are key to the system's continuing success:

- surgeon involvement in all phases of the project
- dedicated ORs for urgent/emergent cases
- clear urgency categories developed and adopted by surgeons in all specialties
- peer review of cases by the surgical oversight committee to ensure consistency and monitor compliance.

As surgeons, anesthesiologists, and staff become familiar with this system, they come to appreciate its transparency, fairness, and predictability. Most importantly, it leads to improvements in patient care while decreasing long days and stress for providers. ❖

—Osnat Levtzion-Korach MD, MHA
Senior medical consultant,
Press Ganey Associates

Kenneth G. Murphy, MD
President, Georgia
Anesthesiologists PC

Susan Madden, MS
Vice president, analytics,
Press Ganey

Christina Dempsey, RN, CNOR, MBA
Senior vice president, clinical operations,
Press Ganey

This article originally appeared in OR Manager, *July 2010;26:1,11-13.*

Managing Urgent Cases with Accountability

A 4-level classification system with built-in accountability measures is used for managing urgent and emergent cases at Munson Medical Center in Traverse City, Michigan, a 390-bed referral center with 14 ORs.

The policy was developed by a steering committee of surgeons, anesthesiologists, OR management, and the administration working with a consultant. The committee started with a 5-level classification designated by the letters A through E but later adopted 4 levels (sidebar).

"As we worked through the ABCDE concept, the committee felt 5 categories made for unnecessary complexity," says Robert Cline, MD, the medical director of surgical services. "Also, from a medical standpoint, we didn't need to split hairs between a patient who needed to be in the OR within the hour and one who could wait up to 2 hours. Similarly, we didn't see a clear clinical difference between 8 and 12 hours."

The committee also did not want the OR leadership to be faced with the situation in which the OR learns of an add-on case at 7 am that doesn't need to bump into the schedule in the next 4 hours but can't wait until the elective schedule is finished at 5 pm. Moreover, the committee thought that if a patient's medical condition would allow a 24-hour wait for surgery, the patient could also wait for 48 hours.

"This allowed the classifications to be functional for us on the weekends as well," Dr Cline says.

How the classifications are used

The classifications escalate as time passes. For instance, a Class B case (4 hours) automatically becomes a Class A case (1 hour) and bumps into the schedule if 3 hours have passed. Similarly, a Class C case becomes a Class B case 4 hours from the deadline and becomes a Class A case if it reaches 1 hour.

"The surgeon and anesthesiologists can review this escalation and modify the deadline if the patient is stable, and they agree this is reasonable," he says. "We rarely need to consider this because we do a good job of meeting the deadlines."

The Class D category is intended to include any inpatient who must have surgery before being discharged.

"We felt these cases were important to allow, particularly on weekends, to avoid prolonged lengths of stay, even if the surgical urgency did not require a 48-hour deadline," Dr Cline says.

Accountability measures

Accountability measures built into the policy are intended to encourage compliance by the surgeons, anesthesia providers, and OR management team.

One measure holds the surgeons accountable for using the agreed-upon classifications. The committee asked each surgical section to define which procedures in its specialty were in Class A, B, C, and D. The steering committee then reviewed and approved the procedures with some changes.

Surgeons are expected to use the agreed-upon classifications when booking cases. They have the latitude to escalate a case to a higher level based on the individual patient's condition. In general, OR leaders do not question the surgeons' assignments of a classification.

"Our staff prompt the surgeons for the classifications and occasionally question a classification if it is not the agreed-upon one," says Dr Cline. For example, the general surgeons classified appendicitis as a Class B procedure (4 hours). One surgeon who insisted on bumping other cases for appendectomies has now agreed that they are Class B.

Being available

In another accountability measure, surgeons are required to be available to come to the OR for Class A and B cases whenever the OR can accommodate them; they must be prepared to leave the office if they need to. For Class C cases, surgeons are expected to come when the OR can accommodate them unless they are involved in patient care activities, such as being in surgery elsewhere or seeing patients in the office (this does not include meetings). If a Class C case has escalated to Class B, the surgeon must come when the OR can accommodate the case even if involved in other patient care.

Staff, anesthesia availability

The third accountability measure is that the OR staff, anesthesia staff, and surgeons must bump into the schedule or call in other personnel to meet the deadlines. For example, if all available staff are assigned on a weekend, and a Class A or B case is booked, the OR management is obligated to make appropriate efforts to call additional staff to take care of the patient within the designated times. Technically, this applies to a surgeon who has booked an appendectomy (4-hour limit) but is involved in another operation that will keep the surgeon tied up

> ## Urgent-emergent case classification
>
> - **Class A Emergency:** Life, limb, and/or sight-threatening condition requiring immediate surgery within 1 hour of declaration and taking precedence over any other case.
> - **Class B Emergency:** Life, limb, and/or sight-threatening case requiring surgery within 4 hours.
> - **Class C Urgency:** A nonlife-threatening condition that may lead to severe complications if surgery is not performed within 12 hours of classification.
> - **Class D Urgency:** Nonlife-threatening condition requiring surgery within 48 hours to prevent severe complications from occurring. Any inpatient case that cannot be discharged until the surgical procedure is performed will be included in this classification.
>
> *Source: Munson Medical Center, Traverse City, Michigan.*

past the deadline; in that case, he or she needs to call in another surgeon.

Together, these aspects of the classification system help keep the surgeons honest in choosing the agreed-to classifications, Dr Cline notes. Escalating levels of penalties are included for surgeons, management, and anesthesia personnel for lack of compliance. Penalties range from counseling to formal letters to fines or loss of OR time. So far, penalties beyond sending letters and providing re-education on the policies haven't been required.

"Our consultant described the process this way—during elective block time, the time belongs to the surgeon to schedule. After elective block time, the time belongs to the patients," Dr Cline says.

"By using the classification system well, we have a system to ensure we meet the patient's needs, at least for timeliness. If that inconveniences the staff, surgeons, or anesthesiologists, that's okay because the system needs to be patient focused." ❖

This article originally appeared in OR Manager, *July 2010;26:13-14.*

Surgical Scheduling: Taking an Important Role to the Next Level

Wanted: Operating Room Scheduler. Salary $33,000

Operating room schedulers reserve space for each surgical procedure in a hospital or ambulatory surgery facility. They determine how long a procedure will take and what staff is necessary. OR schedulers work with anesthesiologists to assign one for each procedure, as well as OR managers who help schedulers select nurses, surgical technologists, and surgical assistants to serve on the surgical team. Successful operating room schedulers possess organization, attentiveness to detail, and problem-solving skills, and the ability to communicate effectively and work as a team. The ability to find solutions quickly when pressed for time is also crucial for the position because emergencies frequently cause changes in scheduling.

This synopsis of job descriptions for OR schedulers posted online highlights the importance of the scheduling function to the OR. The OR scheduler has become a focus for improving OR efficiency, patient safety, physician relationships, and the business of the OR. Attendees at the 2010 OR Business Management Conference in San Francisco described schedulers as "the gateway to our business," "your telephone marketers," "the face of the OR," and "the heart of the OR."

Whatever the title, OR managers are seeing the importance of schedulers and scheduling process to growing their surgical volume and improving OR throughput, and they are working to make the position more appealing.

Gateway to business

"We are going in a direction where health care is a business, and I think it's high time we address it as such," says Bettina Celifie, RN, director of perioperative services, Alvarado Hospital, San Diego. "The OR scheduler is the 'gateway to our business,' and the competition is fierce. We need to reward them for the work they do."

Celifie has redesigned the scheduler's job description to incorporate marketing, customer service, and problem-solving skills and has received senior management approval for a 20% increase in salary to match the intensity and importance of the scheduler's role.

"If we are going to ask for a critical skill set in our schedulers, I believe we have to pay for that," she says.

Celifie sees the best candidate for OR scheduler as a person with a background in surgery, such as a surgical technologist (ST), who has good computer skills, a customer-friendly personality, and is willing to troubleshoot.

She prefers having the scheduler located at the OR's front desk because she believes opportunities for troubleshooting, communication, and marketing to surgeons are missed when the scheduler is at a distant location.

Marketing the OR

Speaking at the conference about transforming an OR into a better performer, Jeffry Peters said, "Your schedulers can make or break your business. You need to have the right person in place, and they need to be customer-relations focused, with training if necessary."

Peters, who is president of Surgical Directions, LLC, a Chicago-based perioperative and anesthesia consulting firm, refers to OR schedulers as "your telephone marketers." An important part of their job, he says, is to grow case volume. "If schedulers make it easy and comfortable for surgeons' offices to schedule cases, they are likely to schedule more." Peters suggested that sales incentives be awarded to schedulers for helping to grow surgical volume. Better performing ORs are considering incentives for all staff, especially schedulers, he says. Examples are free lunch passes, movie passes, and bonuses based on growth in OR volume.

Building relationships

An initiative at North Shore University Hospital in Manhasset, New York, has helped schedulers to increase the surgical volume by informing them of service line volume budgets for the year as well as the volume year-to-date, says Bini Varughese, director of perioperative business operations.

With this information, the schedulers know which service lines are above and below the volume budget and can work collaboratively to get cases booked with the offices.

"Our schedulers are empowered to build relationships with the surgeons' offices and be the 'face' of the OR," he says.

Heart of the OR

The schedule is the heart of the OR, and the scheduler is what makes it tick, says Patricia

4 tips for better scheduling

Standardize nomenclature for all procedures

For example, use the term "Hip, arthroplasty, right" instead of "Right total hip"; "Right hip replacement"; or "Total joint replacement, hip, right." Some organizations use CPT codes along with the standardized nomenclature in scheduling.

Develop a standard form

Develop a form for surgeons' offices to fax or send electronically with all pertinent information. Once the case is scheduled, send a confirmation number to the office.

Provide dual monitor screens

Give schedulers 2 computer monitor screens so they can read the electronic fax or e-mail form on one screen while entering information into the OR scheduling system on the other screen.

Communicate with offices

- Provide in-person communication to the surgeons' offices.
- Hold a lunch or breakfast for all the surgeons' office schedulers and office managers to review scheduling policies and procedures. Follow up with office visits.

Source: Pat Mews, MHA, RN, CNOR.

Mews, MHA, RN, CNOR, management consultant, Scottsdale, Arizona.

How the scheduler enters cases in the schedule determines many things—staffing, case picking, and equipment availability, among others. If a case is scheduled incorrectly, then the wrong preference card will be picked, leading to an incorrect case setup that could compromise patient safety.

Because the OR scheduler is the first person the surgeon's office has contact with when scheduling a case, the scheduler's knowledge of the OR and procedures, marketing skills, and follow-up are what sells an OR. Many surgeons have a choice of facilities and will schedule at the hospital that makes it easiest for them, notes Mews. The scheduler's job is to make scheduling as easy and streamlined as possible.

In addition to the job description, Mews says schedulers should have defined roles and responsibilities. She also suggests measuring performance annually and holding schedulers accountable to their defined responsibilities. Data is key to tracking the scheduler's performance, she notes, and can include monitoring incorrectly scheduled cases or wrong preference cards picked for a case.

With the scheduler's responsibilities and impact on OR operations, Mews suggests that schedulers be paid at least as much as an administrative assistant.

"If your administrative assistants have a starting pay of $15 an hour with experience, then that's what schedulers should be paid," she says. Mews recommends that schedulers be paid $20 an hour after they gain experience and be paid incentives for performance but not for volume.

She prefers to have schedulers located in a quiet office in the OR rather than at another location because she finds the close collaboration with the specialty team leaders and surgeons gives the schedulers a sense of ownership of the process.

"If your schedule is botched up, it's usually by someone that doesn't have ownership in the OR," she says. (Tips for improving scheduling are in the sidebar.)

Target for improving efficiency

Carolina East Health System in New Bern, North Carolina, targeted its schedulers and scheduling process as one aspect of improving the functioning of the OR. The system centralized the 3 OR schedulers to 1 location and revamped the way it schedules OR cases. Requests for case time from physicians' offices are now made by e-fax rather than telephone.

"The old system had a lot of inefficiencies," says Robin Schaefer, MSNA, CRNA, director of perioperative services.

Schedulers were doing double the work needed. They were answering the phone, writing down the request for case and time, looking at the schedule for a time allotment, telling the office secretary what time was available, and entering the scheduled case into the system. Now the request for the procedure is faxed from the physician's office. The scheduler enters the case in the schedule and calls the office to confirm it.

More satisfied surgeons

Another change that has improved OR performance is that most surgeons have a minimum block time of 8 hours rather than 4.5 hours. This change to 8-hour blocks was based on projected utilization evaluated for several months, notes Schaefer. The surgeons who do not have a block had utilization below 65% or do their cases during off hours. Eventually, they also will have an 8-hour block.

Since making the transition from phone calls to e-faxes and from 4.5- to 8-hour blocks, the schedulers and physicians' offices are more satisfied, and the process is more efficient, says Schaefer. "We are actually doing more cases in fewer rooms. With assigned blocks, we were able to close 1 room a day. Utilization has improved overall for the entire OR."

Carolina East holds regular "town hall" meetings, luncheons, and breakfasts for the OR sched-

Patient safety and the schedule

Regions Hospital in St Paul, Minnesota, is standardizing its scheduling process through an automated system with the goal of improving patient safety. The scheduling team consists of field schedulers for each service line in the clinics, and 2 main schedulers who oversee the surgery schedule in the hospital.

Lean scheduling

Surgical scheduling was consolidated into 1 location after a Lean process improvement project 2 years ago, says Dana Langness, BSN, MA, RN, senior director of surgical services. "Before this, we were playing telephone tag between the field schedulers and the main schedulers for the 17-room main OR and 7-room surgery center.

Now the field schedulers who are with the patients in the clinics schedule directly into their specialty blocks in the automated system." If they want to schedule into an open time, they put the cases into a queue and are given times on a first-come, first-served basis.

Because Regions is part of Health Partners, an integrated health system, most of the patients are seen in the hospital's clinics rather than in surgeons' offices.

Reducing risk of error

To help standardize scheduling and reduce the possibility of error, the OR is working with each service line to standardize the names of procedures. After this project is complete, all surgeons will be expected to refer to each procedure by the same name, making the work of the schedulers and OR staff easier.

The automated scheduling system is orders-based with 5 critical components: procedure, laterality, diagnosis, implants, and positioning. These are verified from the source documents.

With this standardized process, says Langness, "My vision is that the surgery schedule will be as reliable as the informed consent."

---

ulers and the physicians' office staff.

"This puts a face to a name. When you know who you're talking to on the phone, it makes all the difference," she says.

Automating scheduling for offices

In 2008, Northwestern Memorial Hospital, Chicago, rolled out an automated self-scheduling system in Cerner's Appointment Book software that has streamlined the scheduling process and increased scheduler and surgeons' office staff satisfaction. Essentially, the process allows office staff to schedule cases directly into the hospital's scheduling system, which are then placed into a queue in the system. Once hospital schedulers review the queue and place cases in the ORs, an e-mail is generated automatically to the surgeon's office staff to confirm that cases have been scheduled.

Before the system was automated, hospital schedulers had a goal to have a case scheduled within 48 hours of receiving the request from the surgeon's office via fax or e-mail. But 36% of the time this process took longer than 2 days and in some cases up to 4 days. Now that the cases are being directly scheduled by surgeon office schedulers, there are no delays.

Productivity gains

Overall, implementation of the system resulted in significant productivity gains for the hospital scheduling department while increasing patient, staff, and surgeon satisfaction, says Arshia Wajid, Northwestern's financial analyst for surgical services.

Before, hospital schedulers spent approximately 6 minutes scheduling a single case. Now it takes less than a minute for them to review the queue and schedule the case. Hospital schedulers and physician office staff specified the information they wanted to see in the automated system that would make their jobs easier and turnaround time for scheduling shorter.

Northwestern comprises 3 facilities, 52 ORs, and 6 OR schedulers. With the new automated system, all schedulers have been consolidated to 1 office.

"Surgeons' office schedulers are very pleased with the new system because it allows them to have real-time viewing access to cases in the hospital scheduling system," says Wajid. Hospital schedulers like it because it has reduced their workload and allows them to spend time on other tasks. ❖

—*Judith M. Mathias, MA, RN*

This article originally appeared in OR Manager, *March 2011;27:1,11-13.*

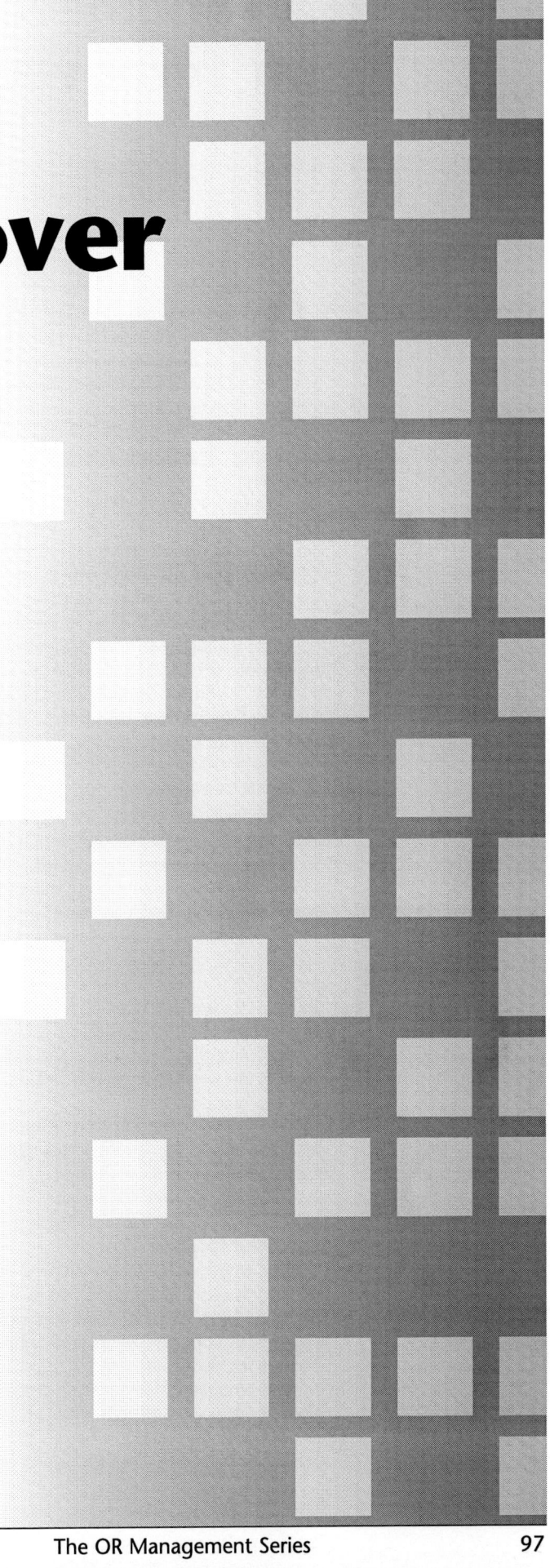

VIII. Turnover Time

An Engineer's Eye on Turnover Time

Airline pilots and race pit crews bring new perspectives to OR throughput, so why not engineers? With the help of a University of Southern California (USC) Daniel J. Epstein Department of Industrial and Systems project, turnover time in 3 California hospitals dropped by an average of 9 minutes, or 21%. The California HealthCare Foundation funded the project.

"We can do more patients per month," says Louise O'Rourke, RN, nurse manager of perioperative services at Riverside County Regional Medical Center (RCRMC), which has 10 ORs and an annual patient volume of 8,824, and reduced its turnover time from 49 to 39 minutes.

From January to July 2008, David Belson, PhD, a professor at USC, and his students worked with RCRMC, Children's Hospital of Los Angeles, and Ventura County Medical Center (VCMC) to improve patient flow.

A fresh perspective

Turnover time is only one aspect of throughput, and it's easy to place too much emphasis on it. Belson advocates a broad view, saying, "The effect of turnover time is more than just the arithmetic of the time between cases."

The OR has categories of personnel and scheduling issues that have to be managed, such as cases added to the schedule, changes in the sequence of cases, backlogs of cases, and the effect of overtime and pay formulas.

Probably the most important variable is the pace of the workflow, which Belson says is difficult to quantify.

"An easy-to-quantify and obvious metric is turnover time," says Belson. "It's been my observation in about a dozen hospitals that turnover time is a good proxy for the pace of work. Thus, if you improve the turnover time, you probably improve throughput."

The engineers collaborated with the hospital staff to examine throughput. "We are efficiency experts," says Belson, who has worked with companies such as Toyota and whose research focuses on health care process improvement.

The engineers helped bring a fresh perspective.

"It was invigorating to have a different viewpoint," says Daniel Ludi, MD, chair of surgery at RCRMC. "They brought a naiveté to the process, and their energy inspired change."

Into the OR

Engineers donned scrubs and spent time in the OR observing processes. "The engineers walked through the layout to see how the patient progresses from point A to point B to point C to get an idea of the system," says Brad Ditto, RN, clinical nurse manager of surgical services at VCMC, which has 5 ORs and an annual case volume of 5,500.

Ditto says for him the reasons for the study were threefold: to add more cases, to decrease overtime if more cases weren't added, and to heighten awareness of staff about how their turnover time compared to that of other hospitals.

"Our weekly caseload has picked up slightly, and our overtime is noticeably down from before the study," he says. "Everyone seems more aware of the need for efficiency, so our turnover times continue to be down from where they were before the study began."

Engineers' suggestions

The engineers developed specific suggestions. For example, VCMC's preoperative area is not close to the OR, and the preop holding area holds only 4 patients for a 5-room OR. The engineers suggested caring for the fifth patient in the postanesthesia care unit instead of the preoperative area, which improved patient flow.

Engineers directly observed in the OR rooms. For privacy reasons, they left when the patient was brought into the room and returned only when the patient left. Through observation and hospital information systems, the engineers collected and analyzed data.

"They broke down turnover time in detail such as doctors, specialties, and types of procedures," says Ditto. The engineers then looked at factors affecting throughput, such as when outpatients arrived at the hospital, on-time starts of first cases of the day, cleaning the room between cases, and add-on and emergent cases, to identify trends.

Devising solutions with surgeons

The hospitals had work to do, too. "We had to flow-diagram everything from mopping the floor to when the surgeon arrived. The process was enlightening," says David Ninan, DO, chair of the anesthesiology department at RCRMC.

The engineers even counted the number of steps people had to take for certain actions.

Having data to present to surgeons was invaluable, says Ditto. "It takes all the emotional aspects out of it." He found surgeons often didn't realize how they affected turnover time. Once they knew, Ditto could work with them to devise solutions. An example is to have a surgeon who simply can't arrive on time for the first case of the day change his surgical schedule.

Staff had their own reactions. When they learned their turnover time was higher than they thought, "it bruised their pride a bit," says Ditto, motivating them to improve.

Engineers in the OR produced a Hawthorne effect at VCMC.

"No one wants to look bad when you are being observed, so staff picked things up a bit," says Ditto.

Achieving better turnover time primarily came through better scheduling, housekeeping services, and staff communication.

Optimal schedule

Belson's team used computer models, including a mixed integer programming model, to analyze data on OR demand for different specialties and OR times to determine optimal scheduling.

"This approach is used by airlines and the petroleum industry to find the best possible way to schedule things," says Belson, who stresses the need to develop a realistic and accurate OR schedule.

He also advises managers to determine their true utilization, noting that hospitals often think it's higher than it actually is. The effort is worthwhile, as OR managers know. As Belson says, "If you don't keep an OR busy all day, you're throwing away a lot of money."

Housekeeping on deck

Ditto says housekeeping personnel are now in better contact with the charge nurse so they can determine workload and schedule breaks appropriately.

The change brought a side benefit. "They stepped up to the plate," says Ditto. "They got accolades and took more pride in what they did."

At RCRMC, the ability to time how long it took to clean a room gave the team data needed to add an additional housekeeping staff member.

"When we have the numbers we can say, 'Yes, that makes sense.' The focus on the data was helpful," says Dr Ludi.

Communication

"Engineers stressed communication, which everyone knows about, but it's easy to forget," says Ditto.

Dr Ludi says RCRMC is adding preoperative briefings and postoperative debriefings in response to the engineers' feedback. Briefings can reduce OR delays. According to a study from Johns Hopkins University School of Medicine, a 2-minute preop briefing reduced unexpected operative delays by 31%. Another change is that "after the patient is asleep, everyone uses first names to promote a team approach."

O'Rourke adds that the team worked on how to use different modes of communication more effectively. Those participating in the project received cell phones and 2-way pagers.

The charge nurse plays a pivotal role, says Belson, and needs to be aware of each patient's status in the OR. "You can use walkie-talkies, a whiteboard, video monitors, or computerized patient tracking systems."

Translation, please

In some ways, the engineers' lack of health care training was a bonus. "To look at our OR through the eyes of someone who doesn't understand the process was a breath of fresh air and renewed our commitment," says O'Rourke, who emphasizes the need to set expectations. "It was very important in the beginning that everyone knew there wouldn't be finger pointing or blaming."

In addition to Dr Ninan and Dr Ludi, the team included Jill Stewart, RN, assistant nurse manager; Susan Rand, DSc, patient safety/compliance officer; and Luis Orozco, LCSW, MSW, assistant hospital administrator.

Bridging 2 worlds

On the other hand, the engineers' lack of a health care background brought its own challenges.

"They didn't understand medical procedures, how in-depth procedures can be and how invasive," says O'Rourke, adding, "We take it for granted. If we went into their world, we wouldn't understand their language either."

Some problems were easily corrected. For example, engineers had to be told that the hospital defined turnover time as beginning when the patient, not the surgeon, left the room.

Other differences went deeper.

"They were unaware of how many factors affect the care of the patient—the appointment, the arrival of the patient, a code on the floor, the admitting process; all those details," says O'Rourke.

Working in a public care facility such as VCMC meant even more issues.

"Our patients have a lot of problems with rides and getting labs done," says Ditto. "They [the engineers] didn't look at some of the inherent problems we have."

Ditto, whose facility was built 50 years ago,

cites the example of the engineers wanting to turn an area into a preop holding area. "They didn't understand that it's not that simple," he says. However, he plans to keep their suggestions in mind if more space or a new hospital is available in the future.

"I thought they were terrific," adds Ditto. "We butted heads a few times, which is good. They validated information we try to give doctors. It's another way of presenting the information, because they were independent auditors."

Do it again?

Those interviewed said they found the experience valuable and would invite engineers into their OR again.

"We want to see where we are," says Dr. Ludi. "It helped us to look inside [our processes]."

If you're interested in an engineer's take on your OR, Belson recommends contacting larger universities, which likely have an industrial engineering or systems engineering department. Fewer than 10 such schools currently focus on health care. But, he says, "Health care is a hot topic these days, and it's going to get hotter. Engineering schools are looking at how to get involved in health care, so schools would probably be receptive."

If that's not an option, he suggests using manufacturing-based training programs such as The Toyota Way (Lean manufacturing) to promote process improvement.

Of course, improving throughput is an ongoing effort, with or without engineers. "It's not just turnover time," says Dr Ninan. "It's a constant process that we're always working on." ❖

—*Cynthia Saver, RN, MS*

Cynthia Saver is a freelance writer in Columbia, Maryland.

References

Nundy S, Mukherjee A, Sexton J B, Pronovost PJ, et al. Impact of preoperative briefings on operating room delays: Apreliminary report. *Arch Surg.* 2008;143(11):1068-72.

This article originally appeared in OR Manager, *September 2009;25:25-27.*

Turnover? Focus on Everything Else

If your OR wants to improve on-time first-case starts and turnover time—focus on everything else. That's the advice of Integris Southwest Medical Center in Oklahoma City, recently recognized as a "leading performer" for OR first-case on-time starts by VHA, Inc. Its strong performance is the outgrowth of a 4-year focus on Lean management, plus a locally developed surgical logistics system.

Byproduct of periop process

On-time starts and turnover time "are a byproduct of the entire perioperative process. You cannot focus on that, or you will underperform in the other areas," says Keley John Booth, MD, chairman of anesthesiology at Integris Southwest and president of Advanced Perioperative Services, PC, who built the logistics systems from the ground up.

Here is his logic. A patient having a routine procedure like a laparoscopic cholecystectomy typically is in and out of the hospital in 4 to 5 hours, or about 300 minutes at most.

"If your turnover time is 30 minutes, that is only 10% of that time. I think you get a lot more bang for the buck by focusing on the 90%," he says.

Integris Southwest was recognized by VHA, Inc, for first-case on-time starts averaging 73.6% over 12 months. (On time is defined as the patient in the room no later than the scheduled time.) Its turnover time for patient out to patient in, averaging 18 minutes for 12 months, is on a par with top performers. Meanwhile, OR staffing costs were reduced by 18.5% on a per-minute basis, and surgical volume rose by 7.95%.

Untangling the process

Before launching its Lean effort in 2006, Integris Southwest faced the same frustration as many ORs. "We were making hundreds of phone calls," says Marva Harrison, MBA, RN, assistant vice president for perioperative/ancillary services for the 10-OR department. "We would pick up the phone on the day of surgery and ask, 'Did this patient preadmit? Are they in a room?'"

Dr Booth recalls realizing during an early Lean event how tangled the process was. "We decided to ask a simple question, 'If Dr S has an 8 am surgery, where is the patient?'

"It hit me that the problem was not that we didn't have enough people," he says. "It was that we didn't have fluid communication among the departments."

The first solution was a rudimentary shared spreadsheet that caregivers could use to communicate about patients' status (OR *Manager*, May 2009, p 16-17, 20).

Technology for communication

From that starting point, Dr Booth, a technology buff, went on to develop the sophisticated logistics software with displays throughout perioperative services. The system can also send messages and alerts to any smart phone with a browser, meaning physicians can access their schedule and any changes from their home or office. The software is owned by his anesthesia group.

Patient status and changes are displayed in real time. For example, if a lap chole is changed from OR 4 to OR 9 or if a surgeon is running late, the change is displayed where everyone can see it. No phone calls are needed. Nurses can enter

Integris's OR performance

	Integris (average)	Proprietary database (top quartile)
First-case on-time starts	73.6%	58.0%
Turnover time*	18.8 min	21 min

*Patient out to patient in.

Source: VHA Inc.

VHA Leading Practice Blueprint™
INTEGRIS Southwest Medical Center - Operating Room Throughput
Turnover Time is a Symptom of all Other Processes

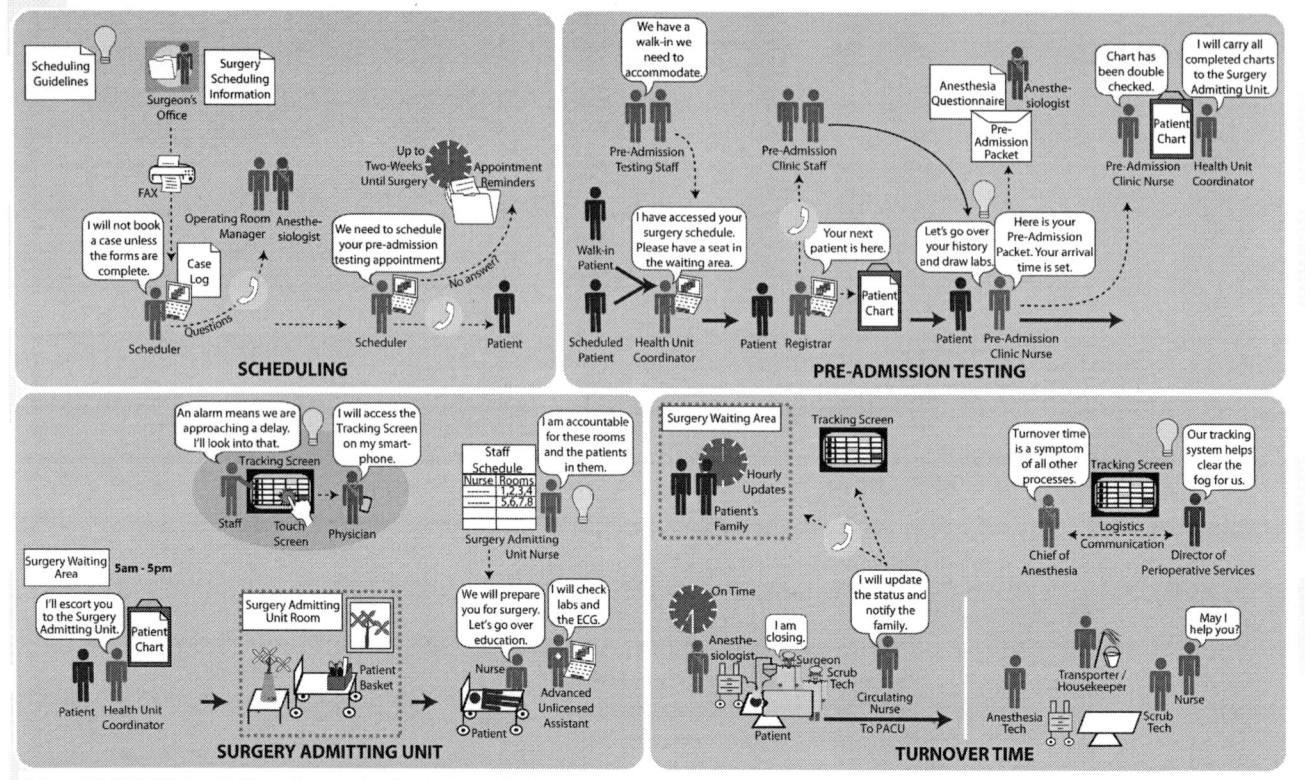

© Copyright 2010 VHA Inc. All Rights Reserved. Reprinted with permission.

status updates easily using touch screens. The software also sends alerts. If there's a delay in preparing a patient for surgery, for instance, the system sends an alert.

"We are in real time able to communicate with our physicians, our day surgery department, and our PACU," says Harrison, referring to the post-anesthesia care unit. "We know where the patient is at all times and whether the patient is ready for surgery."

The software can also produce reports that aid in accurate case scheduling and staffing.

On-time starts

Having instant access to information is a boon in starting cases on time, as are other improvements Integris Southwest has made.

The preadmission process has been fine-tuned. About 80% to 90% of patients have a preadmission evaluation before the day of surgery. That way, charts are complete when patients arrive for their procedures.

Before a case is scheduled, specific information is required from the physician's office, including patient demographics, the diagnosis, planned procedures, and predicted case length to help in preparing the patient and the schedule prior to the surgery date.

Harrison also changed how staff are assigned in the preop unit. Before, nurses took the chart of whichever patient came up next. Now preop nurses are assigned to patients for a block of ORs, just as the circulating nurses are.

"That way, they are more attuned to how those rooms are running," she says. "They know whether a room is running late and when the patient needs to be ready." If a patient isn't ready, they realize they will be identified as one of the responsible parties.

Saving on staffing

Staffing costs have gone down as performance has gone up. Harrison achieved those results by better matching staffing to when cases are actually performed. For example, on Mondays, there is a big influx of patients at 7 am, the pace slows at noon, and then picks up later in the day.

She found when she compared the staffing pattern to that, it was the opposite. "Our staffing didn't follow the bulk of patients," she says. "I might not have had enough staff in the morning. Then a bunch came in at noon to cover for lunches, and many went home at 3, just when physicians were returning from their offices to perform more cases." Reports from the logistics system helps her see when more or fewer staff are needed to match the cases.

Hiring for improvement

Technology alone won't improve performance.

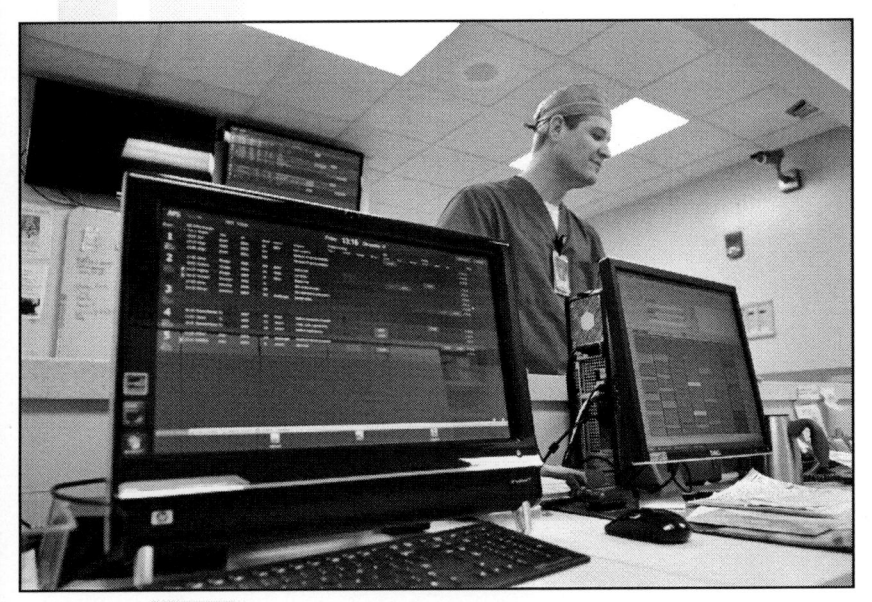

Screens throughout surgical services display the status of patients and related information.

The entire organization, from administrators to front-line staff, have to adopt a culture of relentless improvement, Dr Booth and Harrison emphasize.

That extends to hiring.

"When you want to move your organization forward, you have to hire and train the type of person who is going to fit with your organization," Harrison says.

"We want people who will fit into our culture of continuous improvement. We will never get to the point where our efficiency is where we want it to be—we can always do better."

How do you hire the "right person"? There is no magic, she notes. "We look for people who are excited about the job and don't see it just as an 8-hour workday. Our managers have embraced our culture. They know what we need, and they look for those characteristics."

In interviews, managers ask questions to elicit a candidate's attitude toward performance improvement (PI), such as "What are your ideas for the OR? What can we learn from you?" They watch for signals that the person is not focused mainly on how many hours he or she will work.

Hand-in-hand

The logistics software and continuous improvement philosophy go hand-in-hand. "You cannot get the successes we have without putting all of the puzzle pieces in place," Harrison says. "There are 50 things behind every process we have changed.

"It doesn't work to take one piece of the puzzle, like turnover time. You have to constantly change and work on every process you have."

A hospital doesn't have to adopt Lean management—any performance improvement method can be effective as long as you stick with it, Dr Booth notes.

Adds Harrison, "I'm glad we have Lean at Integris, but we could have picked any tool. As long as you have the attitude that you are going to improve, you can use any tool available."

The physicians are on board.

"It really is the physicians' ideas we work on," she says. "They don't come to me with problems any more—'My case didn't start on time; you delayed me.' They come to me with projects they want to look at."

With the logistics software and the consistent focus on PI, Harrison says, "our cases being on time and our turnover times are among the best in the country. I would put us up against any surgery center.

"And we didn't do it by adding staff or more ORs. We did it with our efficiency." ❖

—*Pat Patterson*

This article originally appeared in OR Manager, *April 2011;27:20-22.*

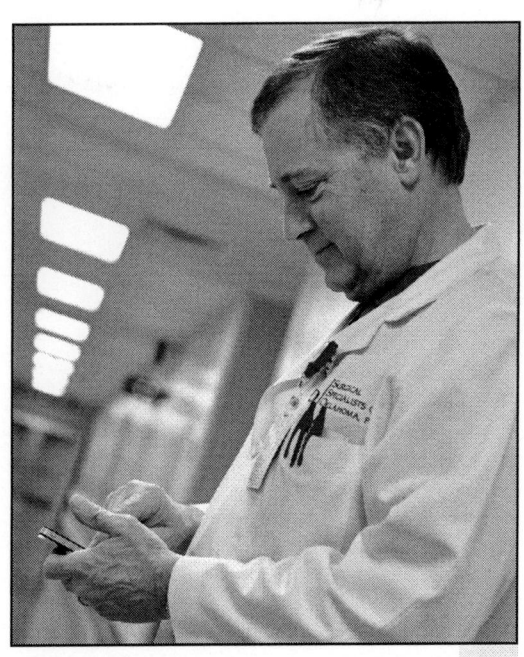

Physicians can access their schedule and patients' status on their smart phones.